POISON

A

HISTORY

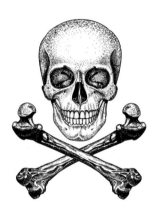

POISON

— A —

HISTORY

AN ACCOUNT OF THE DEADLY ART & ITS MOST INFAMOUS PRACTITIONERS

JENNI DAVIS

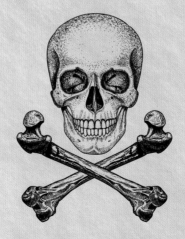

CHARTWELL
BOOKS

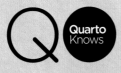

Q Quarto Knows

Inspiring | Educating | Creating | Entertaining

Brimming with creative inspiration, how-to projects, and useful information to enrich your everyday life, Quarto Knows is a favorite destination for those pursuing their interests and passions. Visit our site and dig deeper with our books into your area of interest: Quarto Creates, Quarto Cooks, Quarto Homes, Quarto Lives, Quarto Drives, Quarto Explores, Quarto Gifts, or Quarto Kids.

© 2018 Text & design JMS Books LLP

This edition published in 2018 by Chartwell Books,
an imprint of The Quarto Group,
142 West 36th Street, 4th Floor, New York, NY 10018, USA
T (212) 779-4972 F (212) 779-6058
www.QuartoKnows.com

Chartwell Books titles are also available at discount for retail, wholesale, promotional, and bulk purchase. For details, contact the Special Sales Manager by email at specialsales@quarto.com or by mail at The Quarto Group, Attn: Special Sales Manager, 401 Second Avenue North, Suite 310, Minneapolis, MN 55401, USA.

10 9 8 7 6 5 4 3 2 1

ISBN: 978-0-7858-3588-2

Designed by Chris Bell, cbdesign

Printed in China

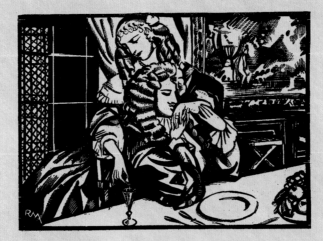

The author, publisher and copyright holder assume no responsibility for any injury, loss, or damage caused or sustained as a consequence of the use or application of the contents of this book. This book describes a variety of toxic substance and none of its contents should be taken as encouraging experimentation with or use of any toxic substance. If you think you have been exposed to a poisonous substance, seek medical attention immediately.

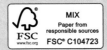

CONTENTS

INTRODUCTION

Poison (noun): A substance capable of causing the illness or death of a living organism when introduced or absorbed.

Poison (verb): To administer poison, either deliberately or accidentally.

(from the Old French for "magic potion")

Oxford English Dictionary

T HROUGHOUT HISTORY, humankind has been acquiring knowledge of poisons and using that intelligence for all manner of nefarious purposes, from disposing of inconvenient people (rulers and relatives in particular) to committing suicide and, more recently, for use as a weapon of war capable of killing vast numbers of people in one lethal attack. *Poison: A History* guides you on a journey through more than two millennia of famous and infamous poisonings, from the ancient civilizations of Greece and Rome to the latest uses in the twenty-first century, portraying the motive (almost inevitably love, money, or politics), circumstances, and outcome of each incident in its historical context—many of the tales are tragic, some outrageous, and a few even border on the comical. And look out for glimpses into the "poison cabinet," which provides brief descriptions of the source of various poisons and their effects on their unfortunate victims.

The timeline begins in ancient Greece with the philosopher Socrates, who committed suicide using hemlock. Suicide is often considered a sin, but in ancient Greece and Rome it was deemed acceptable as a form of self-administered euthanasia, honorable for soldiers on the battlefield who would otherwise fall into the hands of the enemy, and appropriate for criminals. Socrates fell into the latter category, at least as far as the authorities were concerned, and his suicide was state sponsored—or, more accurately, not optional. Cleopatra, too, is said to have committed suicide, but she chose asp venom as her instrument of death. Like many others learning about poisons, Cleopatra carried out endless experiments to gauge their efficacy (or otherwise). Her guinea pigs included hapless prisoners who were already condemned to death, but the poor, the sick, and animals were also popular subjects.

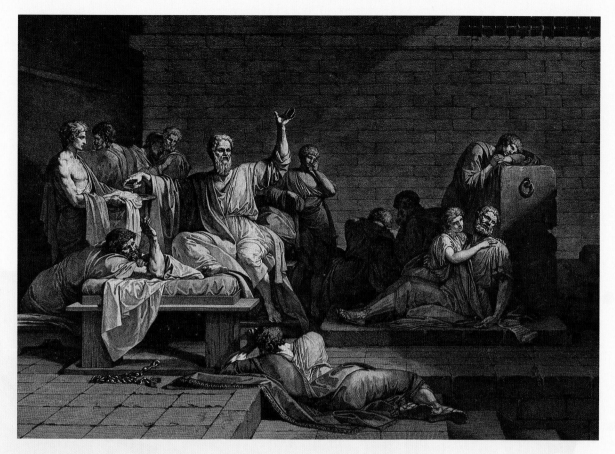

Poisoning was also rife in ancient Rome and reached its height in the first century CE. Augustus, the first Roman emperor, was suspected of being poisoned at the hand of his wife, Livia, and his successors fared little better, living in a city where professional poisoners—often women—could be readily hired. Three in particular—Locusta, Canidia, and Martina—were so in demand that they featured in the writings of the chroniclers of the era, with the descriptor "the Poisoner" added casually to their names.

Fast-forward nearly 1,500 years, to medieval Europe, and we discover that poisoning is enjoying a renaissance equal to that of the arts, although it was looked upon as a rather darker art—that of magic. The royal courts were a very dangerous place to be, and the notorious House of Borgia in particular will forever be remembered for the murderous activities of its members. One professional poisoner, a Sicilian woman, was so skilled in her art that the poison she created bore her name: Aqua Tofana. A member of another prominent Italian family, the Medicis, introduced the art of poisoning to the French court and was suspected of dispatching her daughter's future mother-in-law. In England, where Henry VIII was being thwarted in his attempt to replace his first wife with a younger (and more fertile) model, the servant of the obstructive Bishop Fisher was accused of trying to poison his master at the behest of Henry's mistress. Meanwhile, the world had been opening out; explorers were discovering the Americas and not always receiving a warm welcome from the local populations— Juan Ponce de Léon, for example, found himself on the receiving end of a poisoned arrow.

Suicide by poison. *Socrates surrounded by friends and students in an engraving by Jean-François Pierre Peyron (1790).*

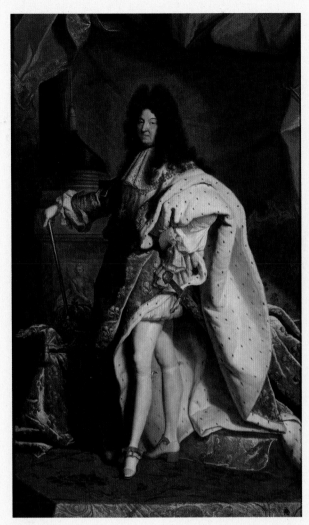

Louis XIV. *His exalted status is proclaimed in this portrait from the workshop of baroque painter Hyacinthe Rigaud.*

The aristocracy continued to engage poisoners throughout the seventeenth and eighteenth centuries, where we find the Marquise de Brinvilliers ruthlessly murdering family members in France. Her trial sparked an investigation that revealed the vast extent to which members of the court of the Sun King, Louis XIV, were engaging the services of poisoners—including the king's own mistress, who had been backing up her feminine wiles with potions to ensure he only had eyes for her. The Marquis de Sade was also fond of aphrodisiacs, which he dispensed freely at the orgies he staged—until he became over-generous with the doses and several of his guests died.

By the late eighteenth century, times were changing. Poisoning was no longer the preserve of the aristocracy, as the middle and lower classes looked to solve their marital and financial problems with the aid of something toxic. And there were other developments—medical evidence was introduced for the first time in the trial of one Mary Blandy, accused of patricide, and the science of forensics was born. Tests for the presence of poisons were developed rapidly in the nineteenth century, tripping up more than one murderer who thought they had planned the perfect crime—Marie Lafarge, for example, poisoned her husband with arsenic, only to discover, to her cost, that a chemist named James Marsh had devised a failsafe method of detection. Mary Ann Cotton feathered her nest with the proceeds of many life insurance payouts before the Reinsch test for detecting the presence of heavy metals put an end to her murderous endeavors. Poison, incidentally, has always been the murder weapon of choice for women, because it requires no physical strength to administer; and a study of poisoners of the nineteenth century found that, statistically, the majority of poisoners were women.

Life insurance was pioneered in the USA in 1760 and the concept was quickly adopted in other countries. It was sold on the grounds that it was the moral duty of husbands to make arrangements to provide for their families should they die; but before long it was seized upon for the rather less moral but useful dual purpose of not only providing a larger income for wives than they had enjoyed when their husbands were alive, but also enabling them to acquire another husband with life insurance, and another…. In the 1930s, the Philadelphia Poison Ring turned finding husbands for predatory wives, and then killing them off, into a lucrative, albeit short-lived, business, and as late as the 1980s, a spendthrift southern belle from Alabama murdered her husband for his life insurance and was well on the way to murdering her own daughter for hers.

Physicians have a distinct advantage when it comes to poisoning, but this is no guarantee that their crimes will go undetected. Dr George Lamson and Dr Harold Shipman murdered for money, Dr Crippen for love, and all three were exposed. Lamson and Crippen were both hanged and although Shipman also hanged, it was by his own hand—the death penalty had been abolished in Britain in 1965, years before the serial killer Shipman ran up his extraordinary tally of murders.

Poisoners have always been very creative in their methods of administration, with food and drink obvious mediums in which to secrete poison. In the Paris of the 1930s, a young girl murdered her father with the barbiturate veronal served in a glass of wine and tried to pass it off as suicide. The English are well known for their love of tea, a fact that Mary Ann Cotton took full advantage of, and as recently as 2006, a Russian defector was believed to have been poisoned by polonium-laced tea in London. But ingestion of poison is not a foolproof method, even when the dose is enough to kill several people, as the would-be assassins of Rasputin, the Russian "Mad Monk," discovered when they served him petits fours generously laced with cyanide and he refused to die; and if the intention was to assassinate the Ukranian politician Viktor Yushchenko with a dose of dioxin, possibly administered via a bowl of soup, it failed—he survived, although severely disfigured. The "giggling granny" Nannie Doss, on the other hand, was taking

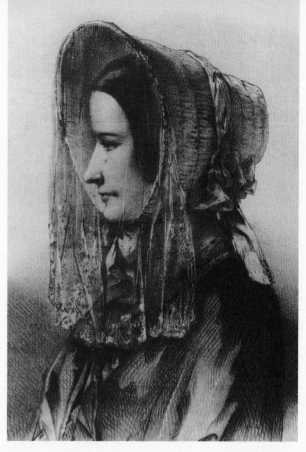

Foiled by forensics. *Marie Lafarge's guilt was revealed through the Marsh test for arsenic.*

no chances and the exhumed body of her fifth husband was discovered to contain a huge quantity of arsenic; and in one of the most bizarre events of the twentieth century, the mass suicide of 918 members of the Peoples Temple cult took place in Jonestown, Guyana, with the victims each downing a sufficient quantity of cyanide to kill them within minutes.

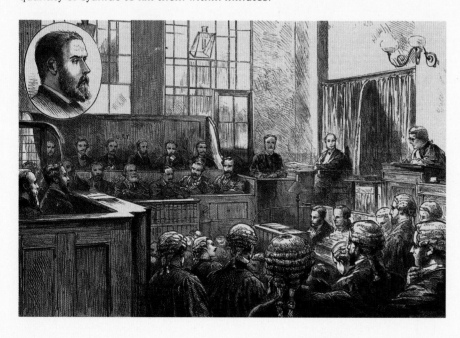

Addiction as motive.
Dr George Henry Lansom was found guilty of poison by aconite in 1882.

Food and drink are not the only vehicles for poison, however, and some murders carried out in modern times have been so bold they seem more likely to be a figment of a scriptwriter's imagination than real life: a Mafia hitman wielding a nasal spray bottle filled with cyanide; a Bulgarian dissident stabbed with a poisoned umbrella; a former Russian military intelligence officer and British spy living in England poisoned by a novichok nerve agent in Salisbury in 2018, along with his daughter; and perhaps most surreal of all, a synchronized attack on the Toyko subway, in which five terrorists on separate trains released liquid sarin from plastic sacks.

The twentieth century saw poison take on a new significance—while it continued to be used by individuals to sort out their marital and financial difficulties (or aspirations), from World War I it became a weapon of war. Hostilities began with a lachrymator, or "tear gas," a fairly innocuous weapon still in use today as a method of crowd control; but soon, newly developed pesticides such as phosgene and Zyklon B proved highly effective when it came to destroying the lungs of soldiers and the mass extermination of Jewish prisoners of war, while the herbicide Agent Orange, used to expose rebels hiding in forests and deprive them of food, would later be discovered to have far more damaging effects on soldiers and civilians alike. Sarin, another pesticide, was not used as a weapon in World War II but has more recently been used indiscriminately in rebel-held areas of Iraq and Syria, killing both civilians and rebels.

With endless legislation now in place to prevent the use of poison for other than its intended purpose, it would seem almost impossible for a would-be murderer or assassin to get his or her hands on a dose sufficient to kill, but as the accounts featured in this book prove—even today, where there's a will, there's a way.

The creation of the gas mask. *Gas masks were developed after the deadly German gas attack near Ypres, Belgium, in 1915, during World War I.*

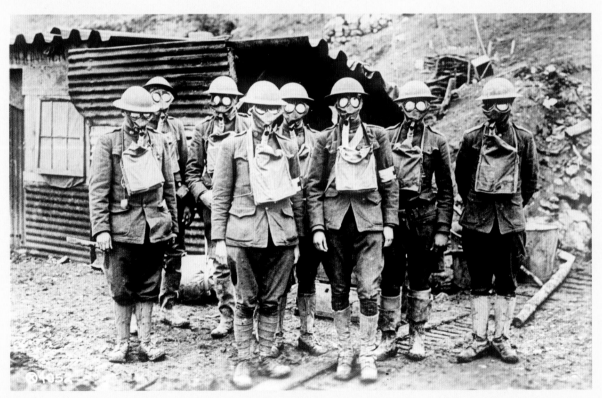

POISONS CHART

Common name	Description	Entry
Aconite (*Aconitum napellus*)	Genus of over 250 species of flowering plants belonging to the *Ranunculaceae* family. Other names include monkshood and wolf's bane	Locusta, Canidia, and Martina; George Henry Lamson
Aqua Tofana	Strong poison based on arsenic, belladonna, and lead	The Affair of the Poisons
Arsenic	Chemical element occuring in many minerals, usually in combination with sulfur and metals, but also as a pure elemental crystal	Mary Blandy; Marie Lafarge; Mary Ann Cotton; Audrey Marie Hilley; The Philadelphia Poison Ring; Nannie Doss
Cantarella	Mythical poison of the Borgias; said to contain arsenic, copper, and phosphorus	The Borgias
Cantharidin (Spanish fly)	Emerald-green beetle of the blister beetle family (*Meloidae*)	Marquis de Sade
Cyanide	Chemical compound; can be organic or nonorganic	Rasputin; The Rev Jim Jones; Richard Kuklinski
Dioxin	Highly toxic compounds that are environmental persistent organic pollutants (POPs)	Viktor Yuschenko
Hemlock (*Conium maculatum*)	Highly poisonous biennial herbaceous flowering plant, native to Europe and North Africa	Socrates; Locusta, Canidia, and Martina
Henbane (*Hyoscyamus niger*)	Poisonous plant in the *Solanaceae* family	Locusta, Canidia, and Martina
Hyoscine (*Hyoscine hydrobromide*)	Medication produced from plants of the nightshade family	Dr Crippen
Manchineel (*Hippomane mancinella*)	Species of flowering plant native to the tropical southern part of North America and northern South America	Ponce de Léon
Morphine	Opiate medication found naturally in a number of plants and animals	Harold Shipman
Polonium	Rare and highly radioactive chemical element	Alexander Litvinenko
Ricin	Highly toxic extract produced in the seeds of the castor oil plant	Georgi Markov
Sarin	Highly toxic synthetic compound used as a chemical weapon	Poisons in Warfare; The Tokyo Subway Sarin Poisonings
Strychnine (*Strychnos nux-vomica*)	Highly toxic, colorless, bitter, crystalline alkaloid used as a pesticide	Thomas Cream
Valium	Medication of the benzodiazepine family producing a calming effect	The Rev Jim Jones
Veronal	Brand name of the first commercially available barbiturate	Violette Nozière

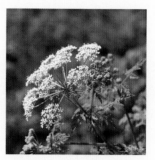

Hemlock

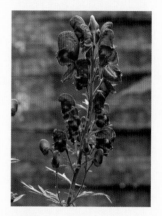

Aconite

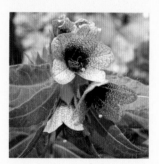

Henbane

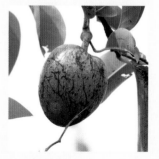

Manchineel fruit

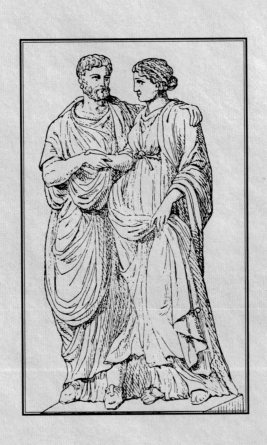

CHAPTER ONE

POISON IN THE ANCIENT WORLD

Humans have invented, tested, experimented with, and deployed poisons for their own purposes for centuries, and this activity shows no sign of decreasing in the twenty-first century. In ancient Greece, 2,500 years ago, we find the philosopher Socrates, forced by society to take hemlock and die a painful death, and then Cleopatra, having carried out a number of poison experiments on hapless victims, choose asp venom as her own instrument of suicide. Did Livia really kill her husband Augustus, the first Roman emperor or is her reputation as an evil murderess undeserved? And just how did three infamous Roman women—Locusta, Canidia, and Martina—establish themselves as professional poisoners. Were they in the right place at the right time or did their very presence spike the prevalence of poisonings in ancient Rome?

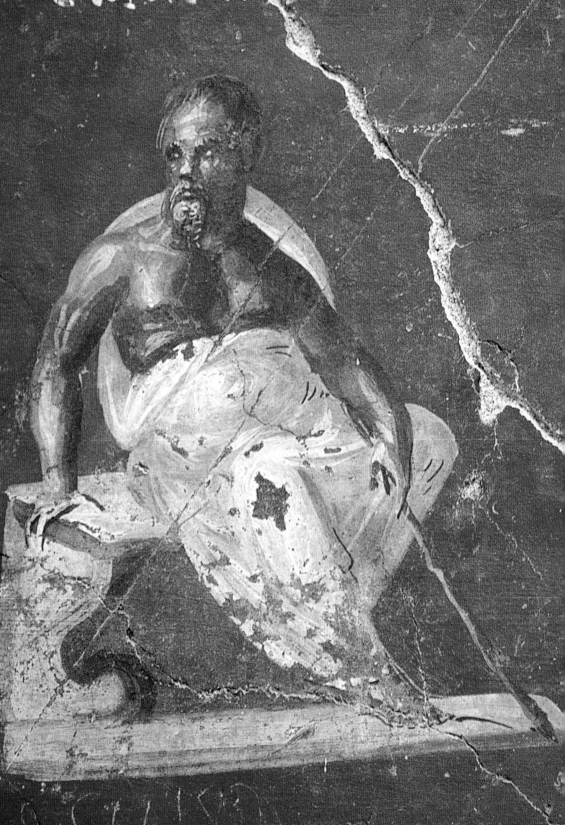

SOCRATES
Suicide by Poison

Socrates may have lived nearly 2,500 years ago but his name still hovers on the lips of every would-be philosopher, so profound was his influence. He spent a lifetime sharing his views with his ardent followers—until one day, the people of Athens decided they'd had enough of him. His life ended in a state-sponsored suicide, and his poison of choice was hemlock.

SOCRATES WAS BORN in Athens, Greece, in around 469 BC, the son of Sophroniscus, a stonemason, and Phaenarete, a midwife. According to contemporary accounts, he was not physically handsome, with a snub nose, a generous girth, and bulging eyes that had the disconcerting appearance of being locked in a ceaseless stare. Despite this (and the fact that he had a keen eye for many a handsome young man), he had a wife, Xanthippe, who bore him three sons. It may be that Xanthippe, like his many admirers, valued his intelligence more than his looks. Today, Socrates is seen as the father of Western philosophy.

A PHILOSOPHER IS BORN

This renowned ancient Greek philosopher was something of an oddball, who in many respects liked to keep to himself. Unlike other philosophers of the time, who traveled widely to broaden their knowledge, Socrates spent his whole life in his home city, except when serving as a hoplite (a spear-wielding foot soldier) in the Athenian army. He did not assert his right as an adult male citizen to attend meetings of the Athenian Ecclesia (democratic citizens' assembly), or attach himself to any political faction; and when it came to religion, he was similarly private, tuning in for spiritual guidance to his daimonion—his inner voice and a gift, or so he perceived, from the gods.

Socrates believed it was the presence of the daimonion—whose sole purpose seemed to be to prevent him from making wrong decisions, rather than guiding him toward right ones—that enabled him to become a true philosopher. Whatever the inspiration, he saw himself as a midwife, like his mother; but where his mother assisted in the birth of babies, Socrates assisted in the birth of the ideas of others, asking one probing question after another of his disciples to encourage them to draw their own conclusions. He became famous

Warts and all.... *Socrates depicted with a brutal lack of flattery in a Roman fresco dating from the first century* BCE, *located in the Ephesus Museum, Selçuk, in Turkey.*

throughout the Mediterranean, and those who gathered to listen to his radical thoughts came from all walks of life, from the highbred and wealthy at one extreme to prostitutes at the other. Some tried to emulate his asceticism, wearing torn clothes and going barefoot. He loved to challenge, to turn ideas upside down, to question the point of something if it didn't bring happiness. "The unexamined life," he famously asserted, "is not worth living." But when he was aged about 70, Athens decided his views were no longer worth listening to.

ATHENS HITS A BAD PATCH

It was now the turn of the fourth century BCE, and Athens was not in the best of moods. Under the leadership of Pericles, the city-state had been at peace following a spate of wars with Persia, and for a brief period enjoyed a golden age of culture. The economy flourished, and with it art, literature, and architecture—the Parthenon was built on the Acropolis, a triumph of esthetics in white marble, followed by the temple of Athena Nike and the Erechtheum.

"True knowledge exists in knowing that you know nothing." —*Socrates*

But Pericles died of the plague in 429 BCE, and the golden age was over almost before it had begun. A new war broke out, this time with Sparta, another powerful Greek city-state, and by the time it ended in 404, Athens was bankrupt, demoralized, and starving. The last thing its citizens needed was more of Socrates' rhetoric (the art that he had learned, ironically, from Pericles' consort, Aspasia); no longer did anyone want to debate "the point of walls and warships and glittering statues if the men who build them are not happy."

The School of Athens.
Socrates is clearly identifiable by his penetrating expression and snub nose in this 1509–11 fresco by the Renaissance artist Raphael in the Vatican's Apostolic Palace.

A CHARGE OF IMPIETY

Socrates was seized on the somewhat spurious charges of "refusing to recognize the city's traditional gods"—his relationship with his trusty daimonion had finally proved his undoing—and "corrupting the youth" (many of his followers were young men). On February 15, 399 BCE, he was brought before the first ever democratic court—three accusers, a 500-strong jury of his fellow citizens, and a huge crowd of spectators—to answer the charges, which took three hours to present. In return, Socrates delivered three hours of oratory. When the speeches were over and it was time for the jurors to place their tokens in an urn marked "guilty" or "not guilty," depending on their verdict, 280 found the elderly philosopher guilty. The jurors proposed the death penalty as punishment; Socrates countered with the suggestion of a small fine. His sarcasm was not well received. The death penalty it was.

SOCRATES' BIOGRAPHERS

Socrates famously wrote absolutely nothing. Everything that is known about his life and philosophy is derived from the writings of others, especially his students Plato and Xenophon. And when it comes to the abrupt end of his life, it is Plato to whom we turn for information, albeit possibly more dramatic than strictly accurate. Plato, like Socrates, was a citizen of Athens, born around 428 BCE to an aristocratic family. He joined Socrates' circle as a young man and some years after his teacher's death he founded the Academia, a college of philosophy that existed in various guises until the sixth century AD.

Plato's account of Socrates' last days falls into three parts, presented as dialogue, a form of literary prose. The first part, Socrates' speech to the court, dripping in Socratic irony, is called the Apology—in Greek Apologia, meaning

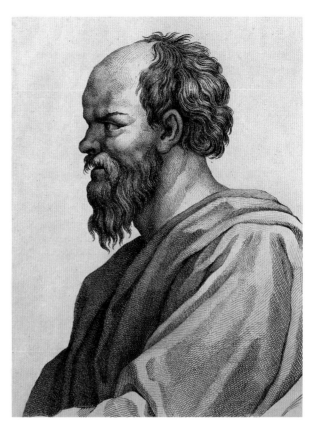

Famous egghead. *This image illustrates Socrates' high forehead, traditionally a sign of intelligence. "The only good is knowledge," he was wont to say, "and the only evil is ignorance."*

DEFENSE OR DEFIANCE?

Although Socrates' speech to the court is described as his defense, it carries more than a slight air of defiance, which was unlikely to endear him to his accusers. And where was his *daimonion*? Why did his divine sign not step in to prevent him making that absurd suggestion about a small fine as an alternative to the death penalty? Had he suggested exile instead, his life might have been spared.

The answer, according to the testimony of Socrates' friend Hermogenes, is that the divine sign refused to allow Socrates to prepare a defense, and that it wasn't in any case necessary because Socrates had no wish to live and had spent his whole life preparing for this moment. He concluded his defense with the words: "The hour of departure has arrived, and we go our ways—I to die, and you to live. Which is better, God only knows."

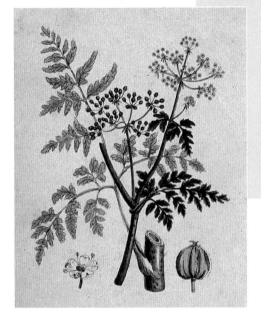

Conium maculatum. The species name of the common hemlock hints at the blindness symptomatic of hemlock poisoning.

POISON CABINET

HARMFUL HEMLOCK

From a distance, hemlock may look like an innocuous wild plant but the purple-spotted stem and fetid smell of the crushed foliage will reveal the fatal *Conium maculatum*, also known as devil's porridge or poison parsley (to which it bears a dangerous resemblance).

All parts of the plant contain, among other alkaloids (substances that have physiological effects on humans), the highly poisonous volatile compound coniine. Consumption of hemlock juice leads to stomach pains and vomiting (a symptom notably absent from Plato's account of Socrates' death, perhaps to spare his memory the indignity), followed by progressive muscle paralysis, blindness, and asphyxia as the motor nerves succumb to its potency. Once asphyxia sets in, death comes quickly. In *Five Little Pigs*, the crime writer Agatha Christie added a dose of hemlock to her victim's beer and killed him off in 40 minutes.

Surprisingly, however, hemlock is used in medicines to treat a wide range of medical conditions—and, even more surprisingly, as an antidote to another poison: strychnine.

"defense." Next comes the *Crito*, a conversation between Socrates and his wealthy friend Crito, who wishes to finance Socrates' escape from prison. And finally, the *Phaedo* depicts Socrates' death. All three dialogues were translated in the nineteenth century by one Benjamin Jowett, Master of Balliol College, Oxford, England.

THE END OF OUR FRIEND

Socrates' execution—which was effectively suicide, since he chose to take hemlock and administered the poison himself—took place 30 days later, delayed pending the conclusion of a religious festival. The *Phaedo* tells us that when Socrates was ready, he called for the man who would bring the hemlock, which had been brewed into a drink, and asked his advice on what he should do. "Just drink it," was the response. "Walk around until your legs feel heavy. Then lie down. The poison will soon act." The man offered the cup to Socrates, who took it without flinching or blanching. Socrates then declared his intention to pray to the gods that his transition from this world to the next should be a happy one, and with that he cheerfully downed the contents of the cup. Those around him were not so cheerful and wept loudly and copiously until Socrates pointed out that a man should be

> "Love is the one thing I understand." —*Socrates*

DEATH BY QUAIL

Most animals have developed the wisdom not to graze on hemlock, but game birds such as quail may feast on the seeds—and if someone then feasts on the quail, they will experience secondary hemlock poisoning within about three hours.

allowed to die in an atmosphere of composure, whereupon they stopped.

In accordance with the man's instructions, Socrates walked about until his legs became heavy, then he lay down and his friends looked on as the poison seized control. Paralysis worked its way up from Socrates' feet, the man checking progress every now and again by pressing and prodding his flesh until it was clear to all that Socrates was becoming cold and numb. The man observed that when the poison reached Socrates' heart, he would be dead. Socrates covered his face, only uncovering it briefly to say: "Crito, I owe the sacrifice of a rooster to Asklepios—will you pay that debt? Don't forget." When the man next opened Socrates' eyes, they were sightless. It was over. Plato recorded, "This was the end of our friend, the best, wisest and most upright man of any that I have ever known."

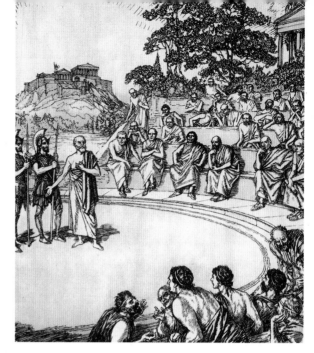

Trial by jury. *Socrates offers his ultimately unsuccessful defense at his trial.*

FAMOUS LAST WORDS

But what of those peculiar last words? Were they merely the ramblings of a man in his death throes? A figment of Plato's fertile imagination? Or, as scholars believe, Socrates' acknowledgment of death as freedom from the confines of his body? Possibly.... Or perhaps it was a very human request by an old man to make an offering on his behalf to Asklepios, the Greek god of healing, who also had the power to restore life to the dead.

Death of Socrates (1787). *Painting by the French Neoclassic artist Jacques-Louis David.*

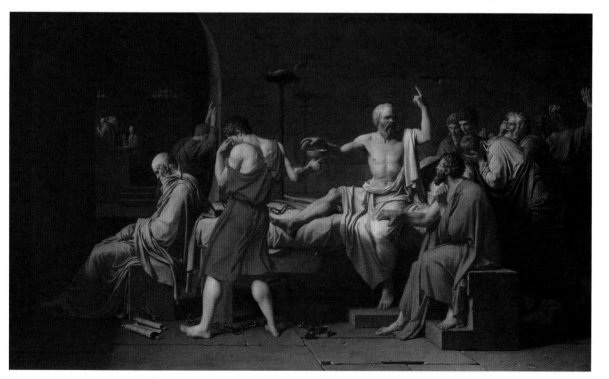

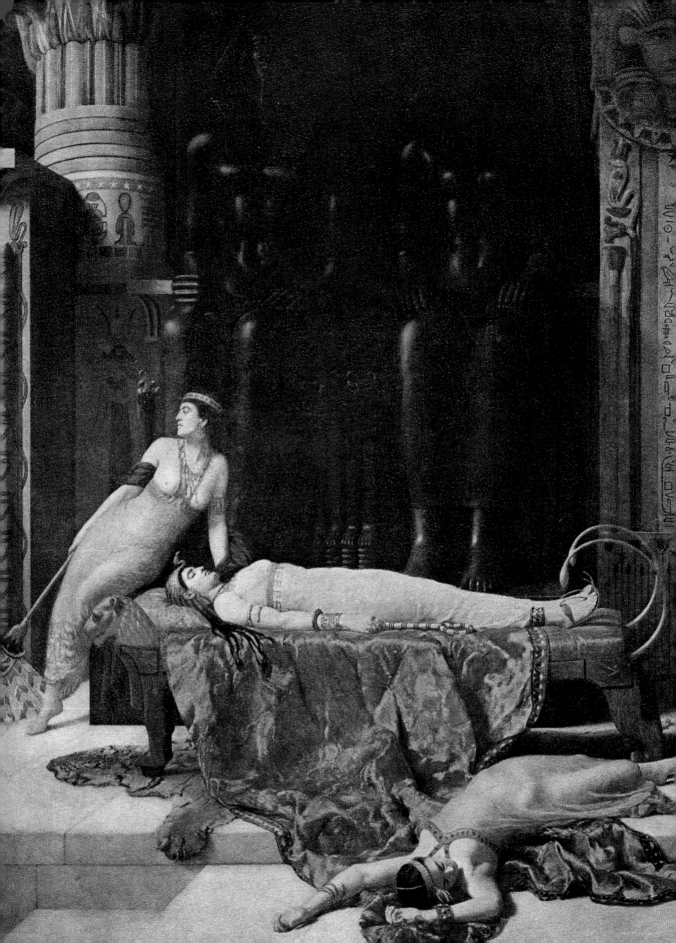

CLEOPATRA
A Nest of Poison

Cleopatra, Queen of the Nile. Portrayed as beautiful, known to be intellectual, a shrewd politician who brought peace and prosperity to Egypt. Loved by not one, but two of the most powerful men of the era. A fulfilling life, indeed—why, then, would she choose to end it when she was not yet 40 years old, using the most bizarre poison imaginable?

VICTIM

Cleopatra VII Philopator
Born: *c.* 69 BCE, Alexandria, Egypt
Died: August 12, 30 BCE, Alexandria, Egypt
Motive: Suicide
Poison: Snake venom

CLEOPATRA WAS BORN around 69 BCE in Alexandria, Egypt, the daughter of King Ptolemy XII Auletes, of Macedonian descent, and a mother whose ethnicity remains uncertain. Although often defined by her power to seduce, Cleopatra was so much more than that—an accomplished linguist, she studied a wide range of subjects, acquiring what by any standards would be considered a well-rounded education.

WHERE IT ALL BEGAN

Cleopatra's ultimately tragic tale begins with another famous name, the Macedonian king Alexander the Great, conqueror and subsequent overlord of Asia Minor and pharaoh of Egypt. When Alexander died unexpectedly, around 250 years before Cleopatra's birth, the vast empire he had striven so hard to amass was once again fought over and eventually divided between three "successors." Egypt fell to Alexander's bodyguard, friend, and biographer, Ptolemy, who became first the country's satrap (protector) and then, in 306 BCE, its king—Ptolemy I Soter (savior). The Ptolemaic dynasty went on to survive (although not thrive) through fifteen Ptolemies, seven Cleopatras, and four Berenices. Our heroine, Cleopatra VII, was destined to be the dynasty's last ruler.

Ptolemy I ruled his kingdom highly effectively from the newly founded city of Alexandria, which he favored over Memphis, the ancient capital. He did not relinquish his Macedonian roots and Greek replaced Egyptian as the language of commerce and government, both of which stabilized as a result of Ptolemy's prowess in economics and administration. Remarkably, although Ptolemy I's descendants ruled Egypt for almost 300 years, they remained doggedly faithful to their Macedonian-Greek origins, refusing to speak the Egyptian language or embrace the customs. Cleopatra VII, however, was canny enough to learn to speak the language and to read hieroglyphs.

> "Poor venomous fool,
> Be angry, and dispatch."
>
> *William Shakespeare*

The Death of Cleopatra. *Painting by the English artist John Collier, 1910. One handmaiden is already dead; the other will soon join her.*

A FAILING DYNASTY

Unfortunately, over time style eventually overcame substance and by the time of Cleopatra's birth, the dynasty had lost its way and was floundering. Some of the empire's lands had been lost to the Romans, and a Roman garrison was soon to be established in Alexandria. Cleopatra, however, was determined to reverse the dynasty's fortunes. She ruled alongside her father until his death in 51 BCE, when she inherited the throne. She was ceremonially married to her younger brother, also named Ptolemy—a move that seems distasteful to modern sensibilities, but in Egyptian tradition a female ruler needed a male consort and the Ptolemies were very keen to "keep it in the family." However, it was not long before Cleopatra dropped her brother's name from any official documents; nor was it long before she began to make decisions without first consulting her advisors—a tactical error, it transpired, when her chief advisor ousted her and replaced her with her erstwhile consort, her brother, Ptolemy XIII.

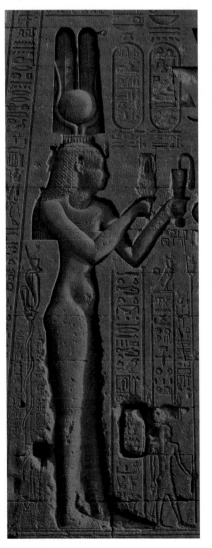

Queen of the Nile. *Depicted making offerings to the gods at the Temple of Dendera, Egypt, this relief is one of the few images that identify Cleopatra by name.*

CAESAR AND CLEOPATRA

Cleopatra's attempt at a countercoup failed and she fled to Syria. It is at this point that Julius Caesar enters the story. In late 48 BCE, while Cleopatra was in exile, busily raising an army to overthrow her brother, Caesar arrived in Alexandria—and Cleopatra saw a way to ensure that she, and not Ptolemy, would be on the receiving end of Caesar's support. She returned to Alexandria under cover of darkness, unleashed her feminine wiles on the powerful Roman general, and Ptolemy's fate was sealed. He died the following year in the battle for the throne. Cleopatra, meanwhile, gave birth to her first child, named Caesarion, whom Caesar officially recognized as his son, and from 44 BCE, having allegedly dispatched her other brother and new coruler, Ptolemy XIV, with the aid of a fatal dose of poison, Cleopatra was now free to govern alone, with Caesarion as her symbolic coregent and later coruler.

ANTONY AND CLEOPATRA

Caesar met his own fate in 44 BCE, when he was assassinated by members of the Roman Senate. From 43 BCE, the Roman Empire was ruled by a second triumvirate (Caesar had been a member of the first). It comprised Octavian, Caesar's adopted son and heir; Lepidus, who was something of a spare part; and Caesar's friend and right-hand

"For her beauty ... was in itself not altogether incomparable, ... but converse with her had an irresistible charm, and her presence, combined with the persuasiveness of her discourse ... had something stimulating about it. There was sweetness also in the tones of her voice; and her tongue, like an instrument of many strings, she could readily turn to whatever language she pleased ..."

Description of Cleopatra from Plutarch's *Life of Antony*

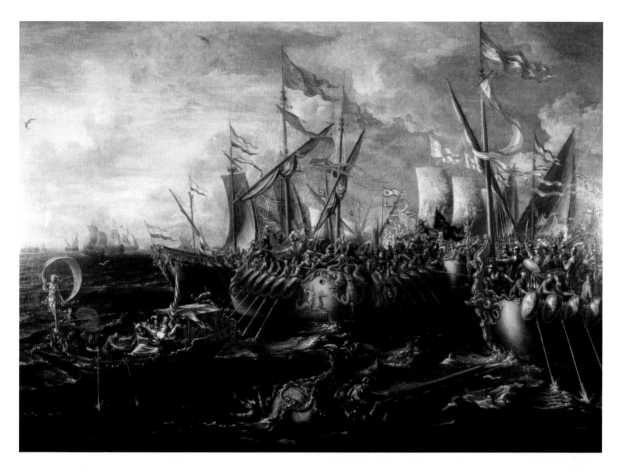

man, Mark Antony. Antony summoned Cleopatra to meet him, and one of history's most renowned love affairs began. Antony spent the winter of 41/40 BCE in Alexandria with Cleopatra, and soon Cleopatra was welcoming their twins into the world, whom she named Alexander Helios and Cleopatra Selene; they were officially recognized by their father three years later. Their third child, Ptolemy Philadelphus, was born in 36 BCE.

The Battle of Actium. *Painting by the Flemish artist Lorenzo A. Castro, 1672. The battle heralded the downfall of Antony and Cleopatra.*

THE BATTLE OF ACTIUM

Antony married Cleopatra, settled in Alexandria, and in 34 BC appointed her coruler of the Roman eastern provinces. The Roman Senate perceived this as treason and a very real threat to the Republic; they recalled Antony to Rome and declared war on Egypt. On September 2, 31 BCE, the combined forces of Antony and Cleopatra were defeated by Octavian's army in the sea battle of Actium. The following year, Octavian pursued the doomed couple to Alexandria. When Antony's forces deserted him to join Octavian's side, he became convinced that Cleopatra had betrayed him in order to save herself from capture. Cleopatra was so afraid of Antony's reaction that she ordered her servants to tell him she had committed suicide. Antony fell upon his own sword and died an agonizing death in Cleopatra's arms.

"Stone dead, lying upon a bed of gold, set out in all her royal ornaments."

Plutarch

CLEOPATRA AND THE ASP

Cleopatra was distraught. Her husband was dead, her own life threatened by Octavian.... She called for an asp, which she applied to her breast. The great Elizabethan playwright Shakespeare puts these words in her mouth, as she begs the venomous snake to kill her: "Come, thou mortal wretch / With thy sharp teeth this knot intrinsicate / Of life at once untie: / poor venomous fool / Be angry, and dispatch." She applied a second asp, this time to her arm, and breathed her last.

According to Plutarch, Cleopatra had written a letter to her oldest son, Caesarion, asking that she might be buried in the same tomb as Antony. Guessing her intentions, Caesarion hastened to her mausoleum but then felt fearful and sent her guards in to her instead. They found her "stone dead, lying upon a bed of gold, set out in all her royal ornaments." Her two handmaidens were with her; one lay dying at her feet, and the other died soon after.

"THE TRUTH OF THE MATTER NO ONE KNOWS"

The account of Cleopatra's passionate relationship with Mark Antony, ending in her dramatic asp-assisted suicide, is so well established that throughout the centuries it has inspired paintings, literary works, and, more recently, movies—but is there any possibility that it wasn't suicide at all? Would a woman so feisty, so independently powerful, really succumb to the easy way out, even in her hour of grief, rather than once again engage her intelligence to take her life in a new direction?

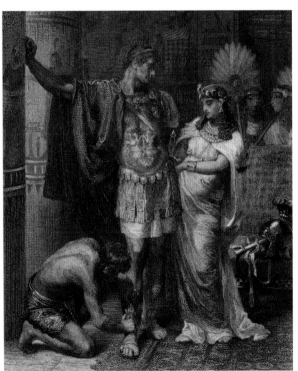

Doomed lovers. *Whether Cleopatra's death was suicide or not, her relationship with Antony culminated in tragedy for both.*

Possibly not, especially given Cleopatra's putative poison of choice. Death from an asp bite would not have been instantaneous, despite Shakespeare's interpretation of events; and in fact there's no guarantee that death would have occurred at all, since asp venom is not necessarily fatal. Someone as knowledgeable as Cleopatra, whose studies had included medicine and zoology, would surely have been aware of this and opted for a foolproof and more immediate poison, possibly the lethal cocktail of plant poisons—opium, wolfsbane, and hemlock—suggested by a recent study. And what of those handmaidens who died at Cleopatra's side? Shakespeare provides one of them, Charmian, with an asp (and instant death), but a shared cup of liquid poison makes far more sense.

It seems infinitely more probable that Cleopatra was in fact murdered by her nemesis, Octavian, who within three short years of her death would control the entire Roman Empire as Augustus, the first Roman emperor. The fact that Octavian had Caesarion executed and then made Egypt a province of Rome would suggest that this, and not suicide, is the truth of the matter.

MISSING TOMB

The only way to establish without doubt the cause of Cleopatra's death would be to test her remains—but the whereabouts of her body are unknown. Plutarch records that Octavian "gave order that her body should be buried by Antony with royal splendor and magnificence," and it is believed that their tomb was situated somewhere near Alexandria. There have in recent years been claims to have located it, but to date those claims have been made more in hope than in certainty.

Cleopatra Testing Poisons on Condemned Men. *Painting by Alexandre Cabanel, 1887. Those already facing death were a target for many poisoners' experiments.*

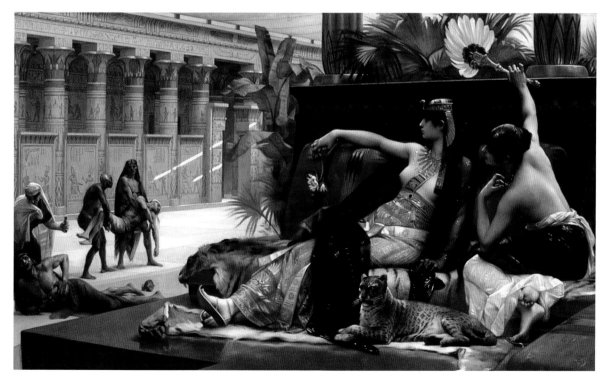

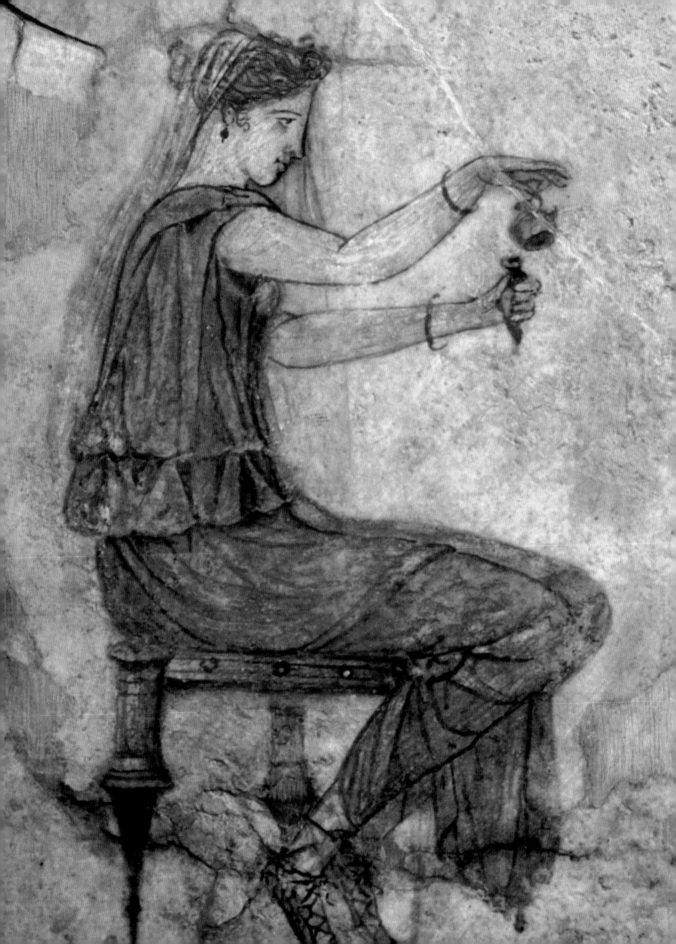

LOCUSTA, CANIDIA, AND MARTINA

Poisoning was rife in ancient Rome and reached its peak in the first century CE, during the brief but eventful reign of the Julio-Claudian dynasty—so what better place for witches skilled in the darker side of botany to practice their lucrative art? Meet Locusta, Canidia, and Martina, Rome's infamous trio of professional poisoners, and their creative recipes for murder.

POISONER

Locusta of Gaul
Born: c. 25 CE, Gaul
Died: January 9, 69 CE, Rome
Motive: Assassination
Poison: Various
Number of victims: Unknown

THE JULIO-CLAUDIAN DYNASTY is the name given to the four successors of the first Roman emperor, Augustus. The dynasty existed for fewer than 54 years, but was full of drama. As with so many dynastic disagreements, it all came down to a matter of succession—who gets the throne when an emperor dies. For those with ambitions to rule, the easiest way to overcome annoying obstacles, namely other claimants, was to organize their demise.

> "A woman lately condemned as a dealer in clandestine practices, but reserved among the instruments of state to serve the purposes of dark ambition."
>
> From The Annals, *Tacitus*

THE DRAMA UNFOLDS

The succession was complicated from the outset because of the lack of a direct bloodline. Augustus himself inherited the throne as the great-nephew and adopted son of Julius Caesar (supplying the "Julio" part of the dynastic name), while Tiberius, Augustus's adopted son who acceded on his death in 14 CE, was descended from the Claudia clan.

Tiberius had a successful military career, but his personal life was troubled. He married for love, but for political reasons he was obliged to divorce his first wife, Vipsania, and marry Augustus's daughter, Julia, a widow with a brood of children, who soon tired of Tiberius and committed adultery. This was frowned upon, and according to a law passed, ironically, by Augustus, Tiberius should have denounced her; but this would hardly have been a wise move on his part. Augustus eventually found out anyway, and Julia was exiled, along with one of her three sons. One of the remaining sons died and the other was killed in battle; and with no other obvious heir, Augustus adopted Tiberius as his son and heir.

Poisoning in ancient Rome. *This first-century BCE Roman wall painting of a young woman engrossed in her task of decanting perfume is reminiscent of Locusta the Poisoner at work.*

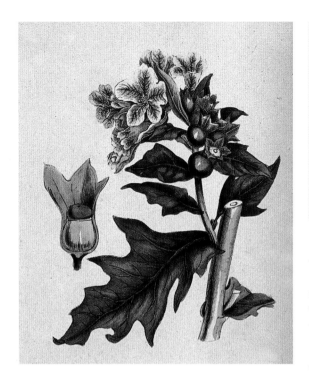

Henbane. *A colored reproduction of a wood engraving by J. Johnstone of henbane ("stinking nightshade"), a highly toxic plant beloved of poisoners in Roman times.*

Tiberius, in turn, had no direct heir, his only child—the son of his first wife, Vipsania—having died in 23 CE (possibly having been poisioned), so he chose as his successor Augustus's great-grandson, Gaius, nicknamed Caligula (Little Boot). In 37 CE, Tiberius was injured in a ceremonial game, took to his bed, and fell into a coma. Death, surely, was imminent. Caligula was sent for and his succession to the throne was announced, only for Tiberius to regain consciousness, sit up, and demand food. This was a hugely embarrassing situation—one that the Praetorian Guard commander swiftly resolved by smothering Tiberius beneath a heap of blankets.

Caligula now held the reins, but not for long. He proved a tyrannical leader and his rule came to a violent end on January 24, 41 CE, when he was cornered and stabbed in a corridor beneath the imperial palace on the Palatine Hill, again by a member of the Praetorian Guard. Exit Caligula. Enter Locusta.

CLAUDIUS AND AGRIPPINA

The emperor who followed Caligula was his uncle, Claudius, nephew of Tiberius. At the time of his accession, Claudius was married to a woman named Messalina, but he had her killed, along with her lover, in 48 CE, and married his niece, Agrippina—who, incidentally, was suspected of poisoning her second husband shortly before her marriage to Claudius, a warning of her capabilities that Claudius would have been wise to heed. Marrying one's niece was incestuous and contrary to Roman law, an inconvenience that Claudius overcame by changing the law. Agrippina had a son by her first marriage, Lucius, for whom she had ambitions. Claudius, meanwhile, had ambitions for his own son by Messalina, Britannicus, but Agrippina persuaded Claudius to adopt Lucius and name him as his successor. Still, Agrippina wasn't taking any chances. Someone had to go. Agrippina's thoughts turned to Locusta.

LOCUSTA

Little is known of Locusta's background, except that she was born in Gaul (present-day France) of peasant stock, became a master botanist and herbalist, and quickly deduced that Rome, with all the nefarious deeds being carried out by the aristocracy, was the place to make her fortune. She was absolutely right, and before long she was so well known for her skill that she was identified simply as "Locusta the Poisoner."

While Locusta managed to dispose, undetected, of quite a few victims, she was twice arrested and twice exonerated through the intervention of high-profile clients; and on the occasion of her third arrest, her rescuer was Agrippina. But Locusta's release came at a price—Agrippina ordered her to assassinate the emperor.

LETHAL MUSHROOMS

The assassination took hours of careful planning. Quite apart from the poisoning itself, Agrippina and Locusta had to consider the fact that Claudius had a personal assistant forever at his side, and servants to taste all his food—not to check that it was perfectly seasoned, but rather that it was not poisoned. Locusta undertook to ensure that the personal assistant was indisposed on the appointed day, while Agrippina would ensure Claudius was in a mood both mellow and unobservant (so that he would not notice the absence of his food taster) by plying him generously with wine. And to make absolutely certain, the poison-laced dish he was served would be his all-time favorite—mushrooms.

On the night of October 13, 54 CE, Agrippina played her part to perfection and by the time the mushrooms were placed in front of him, Claudius was three sheets to the wind. He devoured his mushrooms with enthusiasm, and before long he was showing signs of physical distress—sweating, cramping, and gasping for air. And this is where Locusta really demonstrated her skill and foresight. A physician was summoned, who promptly stuck a feather down the emperor's throat to induce vomiting; but Locusta was one step ahead and had presoaked the feather in a lethal dose of poison. Within moments, another emperor bit the dust prematurely.

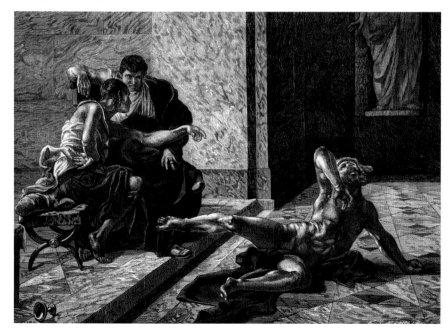

Testing poisons. *This wood engraving, dating from 1876, depicts Locusta with Nero, observing the effects on a slave of the poison she is proposing to use to murder Nero's stepbrother, Britannicus.*

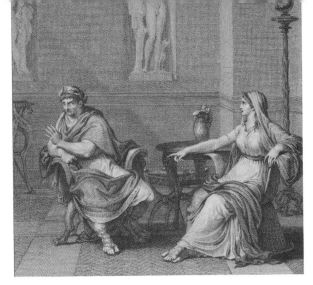

Agrippina and Nero. *"You are an ingrate."* Agrippina reproaches Nero, an engraving from the French dramatist Jean Racine's play Britannicus, *first performed in 1669.*

A SHOCK FOR LOCUSTA

If Locusta was expecting praise and a generous reward from Agrippina for this, her most audacious of poisonings, she was to be horribly disappointed—far from expressing her undying gratitude, the empress accused Locusta of poisoning her husband and had her arrested and sentenced to be bludgeoned to death. But there was a new emperor, Agrippina's son, Lucius (now known as Nero), and it occurred to him that Locusta might prove useful in his endeavors as head of state. He granted a stay of execution and Locusta was, for the moment at least, spared.

LOCUSTA STRIKES AGAIN

Locusta soon proved the wisdom of Nero's decision when she prepared a poison to murder his stepbrother, Britannicus, once it had been discovered that Claudius had named him co-emperor. It didn't go exactly to plan—Locusta's first attempt produced nothing more than an unpleasant bout of dysentery; but a vicious flogging from Nero and the threat of a reversal of the stay of execution inspired her to try harder, and after a couple of experiments, carried out on a kid goat and a pig, Britannicus was successfully dispatched. Nero granted Locusta immunity from execution in his lifetime, rewarded her generously, and insisted that she instruct students in her dark art, so that it could be carried forward for the use of future kings and emperors.

LOCUSTA'S LUCK RUNS OUT

Unfortunately for Locusta, Nero's lifetime was not as long as she might have wished. He committed suicide on June 9, 68 CE—without Locusta's help, although she did prepare a poison for him that he chose not to use, instead stabbing himself in the neck—and seven months later Locusta was condemned to death by the current emperor, Galba. Her execution, on January 9, 69 CE, is thought to have been timed to coincide with one of the many Roman festivals, at which grotesque entertainments were common; however, the suggestion that she was publicly raped to death by a specially trained giraffe and then torn apart by wild animals is thought to be nothing more than a myth. Locusta's name appears in works by the poet Juvenal and the historians Tacitus and Suetonius.

NO RUSH

A poison that caused death almost instantly was not always desirable, and while some concoctions would kill in an hour, others could be regulated so that it took a day, a few months, or even a year or more to bring the unsuspecting victim's life to its untimely end.

CANIDIA AND MARTINA

If little is known about Locusta's life beyond her dubious employment as a poisoner, even less is known about Canidia and Martina. Canidia is such a shadowy figure that it's uncertain whether she was a real person or a figment of the poet Horace's imagination—she features prominently in his works *Epodes* and *Satires.* His portrayal of her was of a woman you would want to avoid at all costs—one who could rip a lamb apart with her teeth, for example, and starve a child to death. He also reveals that Canidia's specialty was hemlock in honey.

Martina is known to have been implicated in the death in Antioch, Syria, on October 10, 19 CE, of Germanicus, nephew and adopted son of Tiberius. Germanicus would have succeeded Tiberius as emperor had he not been murdered; instead, the throne was claimed by his son, Caligula. Martina was held under suspicion of poisoning Germanicus, but she died suddenly, having apparently turned her dark art on herself to avoid being questioned. When her corpse was prepared for burial, a phial of some substance was discovered knotted in her hair, although whether it was poison was never proved and according to the *Annals* of Tacitus "no indications of self-murder had been found on the body."

> "Or has Canidia meddled with this vile food?"
>
> *From* Epodes, *Horace*

It's hard to know whether Locusta, Canidia, and Martina were fortunate to be in Rome when the services of a poisoner were so much in demand, or whether it was their presence in the heart of the empire that made poisoning so prevalent in the Julio-Claudian era. It is certainly the case that far fewer poisonings were recorded once the troublesome trio had themselves met death.

Death of Britannicus. *Nero subsequently became sole emperor of Rome and rewarded his mother's efforts to help him rule by murdering her—but without Locusta's help.*

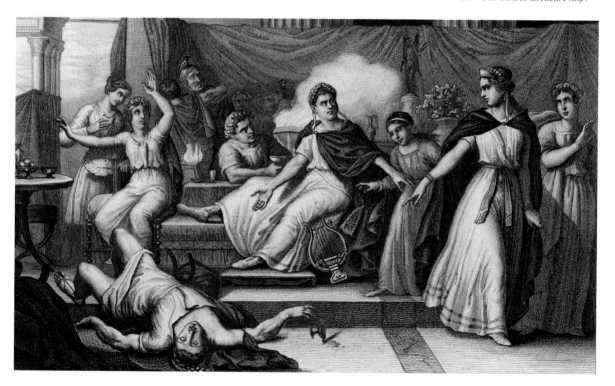

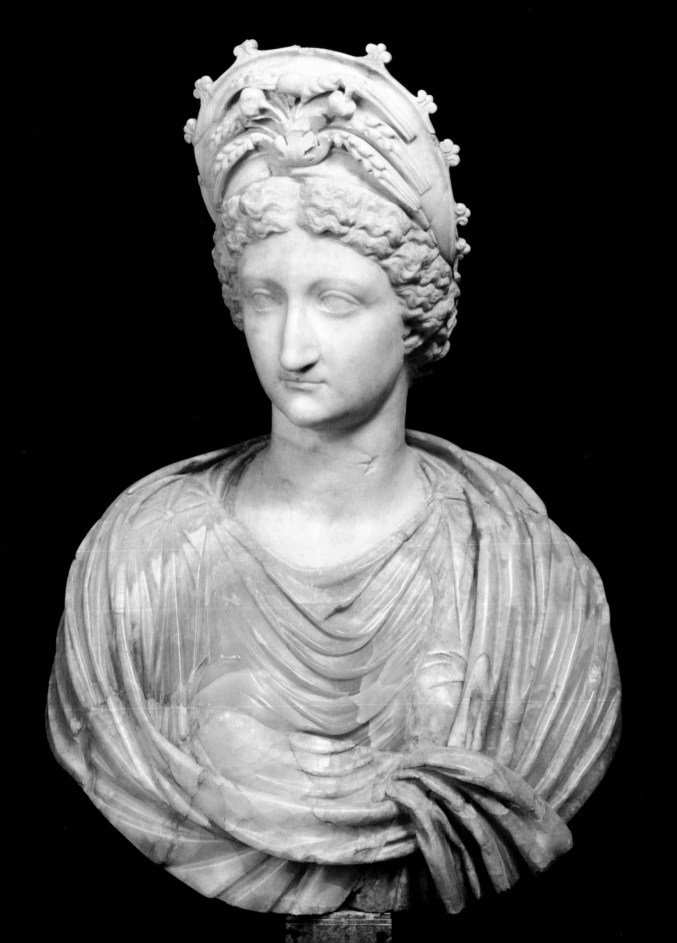

LIVIA

A Reputation Wrecked by Time

In her day, Livia, wife of Augustus, emperor of Rome, was regarded as embodying most of the virtues of the upstanding Roman matron. She was a loyal partner to her husband and, despite his numerous infidelities, they enjoyed a long and apparently affectionate marriage—indeed, many said that she was the only woman he ever really loved.

POISONER

Livia Drusilla
Born: January 30, 58 BCE
Died: September 28, 29 CE
Motive: To gain increased political influence
Poison: Unknown
Number of victims: 1 (possibly up to 5 more)

L IVIA'S HOME, the true power center of the Roman woman, seems to have been run like clockwork. The Roman writer Suetonius recorded that when Augustus died, "he expired suddenly, amidst the kisses of Livia." It was the kind of emotional parting that might be expected at the end of a partnership that had lasted for over 50 years.

So how has history transformed this calm domestic goddess into the calculating poisoner of legend, alleged murderess of the husband she supported through thick and thin? Was she an extraordinarily talented dissembler, or did the Roman historians malign her?

THE LOVE MATCH

Neither Livia nor Augustus (or Octavian as he was known before he became emperor in 27 BCE) was each other's first partner. Livia, the aristocratic granddaughter of a Roman tribune, was married to her first cousin Tiberius Claudius Nero at the age of about 15 and a year later bore him a son, who would become the emperor Tiberius; Augustus was also married, to Scribonia, his second wife.

The years after the murder of Julius Caesar were turbulent for Rome, and Livia's father and husband were on the side that opposed Augustus. The young couple moved from pillar to post, at various points living in both Greece and Sicily, but in 39 BCE an amnesty brought a temporary peace between the factions and Livia, pregnant with her second child, returned to Rome with her husband, where they were introduced to Augustus. On his side, it seems to have been a *coup de foudre*—historical accounts claim that he fell instantly in love with her. And while divorce was not uncommon in ancient Rome, the arrangements that

> "Terrible to the State as a mother, terrible to the house of the Caesars as a stepmother."
>
> *Tacitus, writing about Livia, in* The Annals, *Book I*

Empress Livia. *Depicted as benign and dignified, as befitted her role as first Roman empress. Her headdress bears ears of corn and pomegranates, both traditional symbols of plenty.*

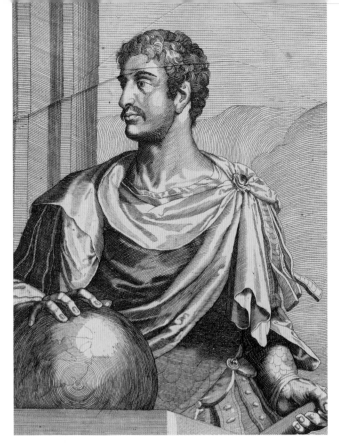

Emperor Augustus. *He prided himself on plain living and plain speaking, but Augustus had trouble managing his large family, who were often at loggerheads with each other. He believed, however, that he could rely on Livia's loyalty and discretion.*

followed were indecorously quick even by the standards of the day. "Caesar," wrote the historian Tacitus, "with desire for her person, wrested her from her marriage." Poor Scribonia found herself divorced on the very same day that she gave birth to Julia, her daughter by Augustus, while the divorce between Tiberius Claudius Nero and Livia took place shortly before the latter gave birth to Drusus, their second child. Augustus and Livia were married just three days after the birth; Tiberius Claudius Nero, whether willingly or not, gave the bride away.

Despite its unconventional start the marriage lasted, although Livia failed in one crucial duty of the good Roman wife—she and Augustus had no children together. Nevertheless, their domestic felicity was almost comically ideal. She was an excellent housekeeper, who oversaw every aspect of the way in which the home was managed. Augustus preferred to wear homespun robes, rather than finer cottons or silks, so Livia produced all his clothes—no small matter when this meant spinning and weaving the woolen cloth, as well as sewing it. He liked her to sit at her spinning wheel in the entrance hall of their house on the Palatine Hill so that visitors could admire the very model of a virtuous wife. She ensured he was fed with plain but excellent food, and kept her own recipes for everything from toothpaste and cough syrup to salves for curing aches and pains. Not only did she keep an immaculate home, but she was also enthusiastic about good works, restoring many monuments in Rome that had fallen into disrepair. For his part, when not at war or on state business, Augustus enjoyed fishing or playing mild gambling games at home with friends. And despite his very definite eye for the ladies (there were scandalous contemporary anecdotes of married women to whom he took a fancy disappearing from the table in the middle of dinner only to return an hour or so later, with flushed cheeks and disordered hair), the couple seemed happy together. Augustus was regularly heard to say that Livia was more beautiful than any of the other women he had slept with.

So much for their home life. As they had no direct heirs, the question of who would succeed Augustus remained open—and a number of possible candidates died young. In particular, two of the sons of Julia, Augustus's grandsons, succumbed rapidly in succession, one possibly from a war wound, the other from a fever. Eventually Livia's son Tiberius would be forced to marry Julia, and would

I, CLAUDIUS
Over 2,000 years after the event, English poet and classical scholar Robert Graves would write I, *Claudius*, a novel drawing on the writings of the Roman historians, which would again cast Livia as a breathtakingly wicked schemer and serve her up to a new audience—who happily swallowed the story when it was turned into the most successful television series of the 1970s.

POISON CABINET

Poisoning was not unusual in ancient Rome; according to contemporary historians it reached near-epidemic proportions during the first imperial dynasty—that is, from the start of the reign of Augustus in 29 BCE until the suicide of the emperor Nero in 68 CE.

Roman knowledge of toxins seems to have been rather hit or miss, although contemporary physicians were on relatively sure ground when it came to poisons extracted from plants. They believed, correctly, that strong poisons could be distilled from yew, hemlock, crocus, and deadly nightshade, but were less reliable when it came to animal substances. Both bull's blood and the extracted organs of certain lizards, for example, were believed to be highly toxic, but today would be held harmless, if no doubt unpleasant to swallow.

Which poison would Livia have chosen to smear on those figs? While they were trashing her reputation, sadly neither Tacitus nor Dio Cassius thought to fill in the details.

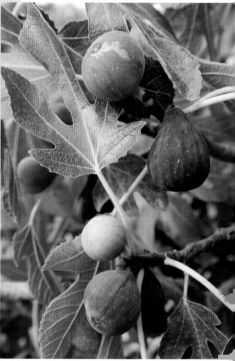

Ficus carica. *The common fig tree was said to be the means by which Livia murdered Augustus. Yet contemporaries described the couple clinging together affectionately as he died, expressing their love for one another.*

then be declared the emperor's heir—and Livia may well have schemed, like any ambitious mother, to help this happen. It would be the historian Tacitus, writing over a century and a half after her death, who would allege that she had gone rather further. Tacitus was a master of implication, all his accusations are carefully set about with "it is said…" and "people whispered…," but he was blunt about what he thought of Livia, that she had murdered anyone who stood in her son's way.

But it was another historian, Dio Cassius, in the third century, who was the first to mention the figs. Like most powerful men of his day, Emperor Augustus was paranoid about attempts to poison him and had tasters who would try all his food before he ate it. Augustus was old and failing when Livia poisoned him, Dio Cassius wrote; Augustus had recently visited Postumus, his only surviving grandson, who was out of favor and living in exile, and Livia feared that the visit would result in a pardon for the boy, and the displacement of Tiberius as heir. So she found an ingenious way to see Augustus off. She smeared poison on the figs of a tree growing in the courtyard, leaving some untouched, then joined Augustus in eating them, taking only the innocent fruit for herself.

Was it true? Almost certainly not, but the tale was too good to pass unrepeated, and the reputation of Livia as an evil, duplicitous murderess was set in stone.

END OF AN ERA

LIvia lived on for 15 years after Augustus's death. Her relationship with her son Tiberius, the new emperor, was poor. He had been forced to divorce his beloved first wife to marry Julia, and he seems to have built up a resentment against his mother in consequence. Poor Livia—upon hearing of her death, he was so slow to return to Rome that her body began to rot and the funeral had to take place in his absence. Not only that, but he denied her the standard honor of deification—a job left for her grandson Claudius, who finally declared her a goddess in 42 CE.

> "Goodbye, Livia; remember our marriage!"
>
> *Augustus, on his deathbed*

Livia **35**

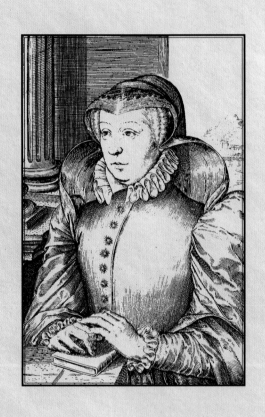

CHAPTER TWO

CASES FROM MEDIEVAL TIMES & THE RENAISSANCE

In medieval Europe poison enjoyed its own renaissance, as a dark art and as life in royal courts became particularly perilous. Catherine de Medici is thought to have employed poisoned gloves to dispatch her daughter's future mother-in-law, and machinations at the court of Henry VIII led to the suspect in a poison plot—the cook, Richard Roose—being cooked in a pot himself. The very name Borgia still has the power to send shivers down the spine, with tales of nefarious deeds. And far beyond the courts, in the Americas, the European explorer Juan Ponce de Léon fell victim to an arrow tipped with toxic manchineel sap, poisoned by those he sought to conquer, his search for the fountain of youth prematurely halted.

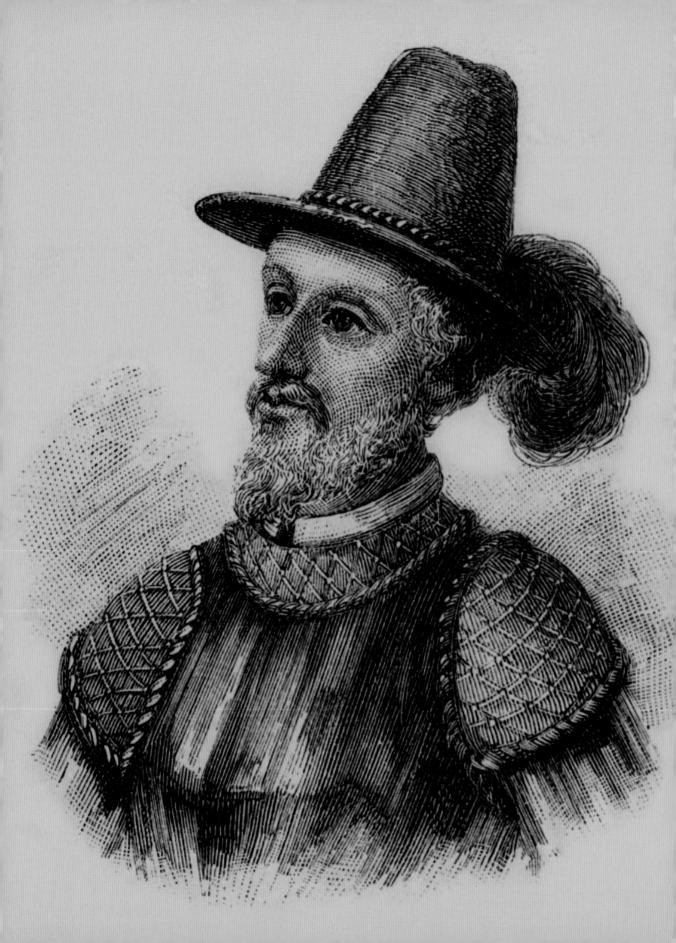

JUAN PONCE DE LÉON
and the Poisoned Arrow

Juan Ponce de Léon lived in one of the most exciting times in history, when European explorers were discovering the Americas. Ponce de Léon himself made quite a few discoveries, and most important of all was the one he made shortly before he took his last breath—that upsetting the inhabitants of this enticing New World could get you shot with a poisoned arrow....

PONCE DE LÉON was born to noble parents in Santervás de Campos, a town in the region of Castile-Léon, northwestern Spain. He fought in the military campaign to reclaim the kingdom of Granada from Moorish rule, but before that he had served as a page to his relative Pedro Núñez de Guzmán, a courtier of King Ferdinand and Queen Isabella—the sponsors of Christopher Columbus's voyages of discovery.

PONCE DE LÉON, CONQUISTADOR

It is thought that Juan Ponce de Léon joined Columbus's second expedition to the New World, setting sail from the Spanish port of Cádiz in September 1493. Columbus's discovery of America on the first voyage had been the result of a happy accident (he was actually heading for Asia), but, armed as he now was with knowledge of an exciting New World to explore, this expedition was highly organized, with at least 17 ships carrying well over a thousand men, as well as livestock and equipment. The aim was to start settling these lands, which were new to the Europeans but not, as the explorers soon discovered, to everyone.

What is known for certain is that Ponce de Léon became a *conquistador*, or conqueror. In 1502, he was in the West Indies, serving under Nicolás de Ovando, the governor of Hispaniola. This was the island Columbus had discovered and claimed on his first voyage in 1492, and which Ponce de Léon had helped settle. In 1504, he was appointed provincial governor of the eastern part of the island. His career was flourishing; on a visit to Spain, he married an innkeeper's daughter named Leonora, with whom he would have four children. In 1507, he was appointed lieutenant governor of the newly conquered chiefdom of Higüey in what is now the Dominican Republic, where he built a house to accommodate his growing

> "Spanish civilization crushed the Indian."
>
> *Francis Parkman, historian*

Juan Ponce de Léon. *The conquistador is portrayed in a late-nineteenth-century engraving.*

A USEFUL SOURCE OF POISON

Europeans in the Middle Ages were very fond of poison and had extensive knowledge of all manner of toxic substances. But they did not hold the monopoly—the indigenous peoples of the Americas were also au fait with the subject, and now that they were being invaded their knowledge was proving very useful. There is evidence that toxins were derived from all manner of sources (including the meat of a poisonous blue otter), for use in hunting and warfare and even in medicines; but the inhabitants of the Caribbean, South Florida, Central America, and northern South America needed to look no further than the manchineel tree, which thrived in the sandy soils and mangroves of those regions.

Today, the manchineel is the most toxic tree in North America but, despite its inherently unsociable nature, it is actually useful, helping prevent coastal erosion via its extensive root system. There its environmental altruism ends, however; its milky sap damages whatever it comes into contact with. Every part of the tree is toxic and potentially lethal—so much so that they sport "Do not touch" warning signs. The sap causes blistering to the skin, and can cause acute keratoconjunctivitis, resulting in temporary blindness. Sawdust and wood smoke from the tree burn the skin, the eyes, and the lungs. It's a tree to admire from a safe distance.

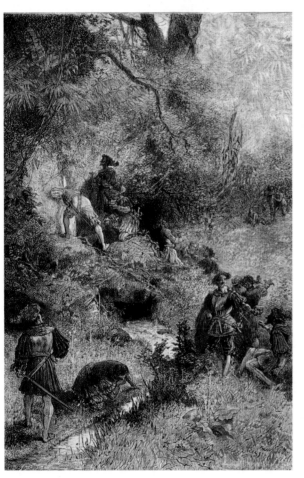

Fountain of Youth. *A woodcut of a nineteenth-century illustration depicting Ponce de Léon's expedition in search of the elusive fountain of youth.*

family. The house still stands today, maintained as a museum displaying items believed to have belonged to him. The estate was lucrative, and the proceeds helped fund the conquistador's later expeditions.

In 1508, Ponce de Léon set off to explore Puerto Rico in search of gold, and founded the first European settlement there. He was appointed governor of the island, and although he later lost the position to a rival, it really didn't matter, because he had the full support of the Spanish crown and was encouraged to continue his exploration of the area. Things were going very well for the intrepid conquistador.

THE FOUNTAIN OF YOUTH

Legend has it that Ponce de Léon now learned of the existence of a Bahaman island called Bimini, upon which there was said to be a fountain of youth whose waters miraculously rejuvenated those who drank them. Whether the story of Ponce de Léon's search for the fountain is as fabled as the fountain itself is unclear, but in 1513 he set off for Bimini. But instead of the fountain, he stumbled on another, far more significant treasure—the landmass of North America, and so it was that Ponce de Léon was the first European to set foot on the North American mainland. However, he believed he had discovered yet another island and named the region "Florida," and the following year was granted permission to colonize both Florida and Bimini.

A LOVE/HATE RELATIONSHIP

In the 1493 Columbus Letter, penned by the explorer to announce the success of his voyage to the "Indies" (which of course was not true—he'd mistaken the Bahamas for his intended destination), he described his first encounters with the indigenous peoples in effusive terms. "They are … so generous with what they possess," he gushed, "that no one who had not seen it would believe it. … They … show so much love that they would give their very hearts."

It was not long, however, before he was disillusioned. The inhabitants quickly recognized the explorers as invaders to be feared, and responded accordingly with hostility. On Columbus's first voyage, for example, he had set up a stockade on Hispaniola, with the help of an obliging local chief, and posted a garrison of 39 men; when he returned on his second voyage, he discovered the stockade in ruins and all the men massacred. It was to become an all too familiar pattern as the Europeans settled the region. Although Ferdinand and Isabella had cautioned the explorers to treat the indigenous peoples with respect, in reality they were used for slave labor and, worse, fell victim to diseases introduced by the European settlers, such as smallpox and measles, with fatal consequences. Retaliation was only to be expected.

A POISONED ARROW

Ponce de Léon was not unfamiliar with dealing with hostility—indeed, he had gained his provincial governorship of Hispaniola in recognition for suppressing a mutiny staged in response to a massacre of the Taíno on the island in 1503. But when he sailed for Florida in 1521 and landed near Charlotte Harbor, it was the indigenous people who held the power. Ponce de Léon and his fellow expedition members were industriously planning the first European settlement on the mainland when they were attacked by the local Calusa tribe, whose ancestors had settled the region thousands of years earlier. The area was rich in flora and fauna, and the Calusa hunted and gathered and fished; by the time the Europeans turned up, they were using sea shells to make tools and weapons, jewelry and ornaments. Life was good, and Ponce de Léon was a threat. "Calusa" means "fierce people," and on this occasion, they expressed their fierceness with a barrage of poisoned arrows—one of which struck Ponce de Léon in the thigh.

THE FOUNTAIN OF YOUTH DRIES UP

Juan Ponce de Léon will forever be associated with the legendary fountain of youth on Bimini, but eternal youth was not to be his. When the poisoned arrow struck his leg, the expedition was abandoned and Ponce de Léon was taken to Havana, Cuba, where he died soon afterward. In 1559, he was buried in the crypt of San José Church in Old San Juan on Puerto Rico, and in 1836 his remains were exhumed and reburied in the rather more grand Cathedral of San Juan Bautista. He would be proud to know that Puerto Rico's third largest city is named in his honor: Ponce.

POISON CABINET
DEATH BY LITTLE GREEN APPLE

Although Ponce de Léon probably fell victim to an arrow tipped with toxic manchineel sap, he would have fared no better had the Calusa offered him a sweet-tasting apple from the tree. Even a nibble of the flesh results in abdominal pain, vomiting, internal bleeding, damage to the intestinal tract, blistering around the mouth, and an excruciating lump in the throat; a feast on the fruit may well lead to coma, followed by death. Its Latin name is *Hippomane mancinella*—"little apple that makes horses mad"—but the Spanish conquistadors named it *manzanilla de la muerta*: little apple of death.

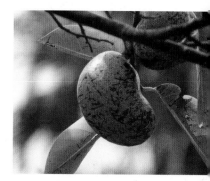

The fruit of the manchineel. *"Little apple of death."*

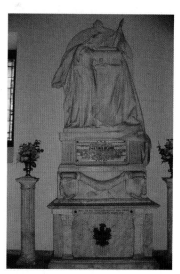

Grand memorial. *The marble tomb of Ponce de Léon in the Cathedral of San Juan Bautista.*

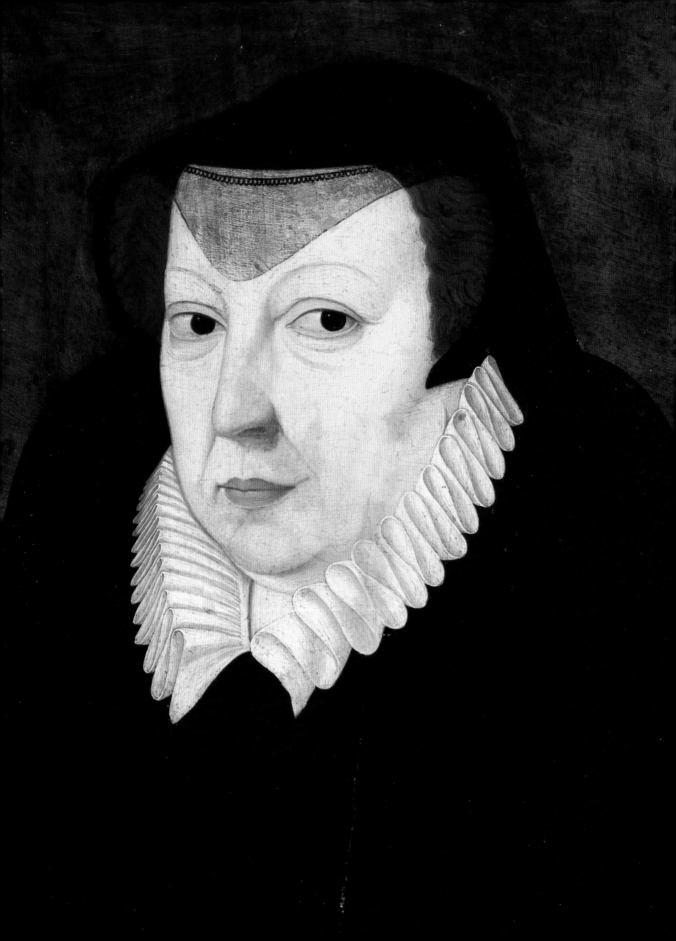

CATHERINE DE' MEDICI
and the Poisoned Gloves

Catherine de' Medici gave birth to three kings of France, found a solution to the French Wars of Religion, and even turned her hand to architecture. There was just one thing to bear in mind about this energetic queen—if she gifted you a pair of gloves, it was best to accept them politely but not to wear them, lest they were infused with poison....

CATHERINE WAS BORN in 1519 to the powerful and aristocratic de' Medici family. Her father was Lorenzo di Piero de' Medici, Duke of Urbino, ruler of Florence, and her mother a Bourbon princess, Madeleine de La Tour d'Auvergne. Within a month of her birth, both Catherine's parents were dead, leaving her to be educated by nuns; and in 1533 her uncle, Pope Clement VII, married her off, at the age of 14, to Henry, Duke of Orléans.

CATHERINE, QUEEN CONSORT

Henry was the second son of Francis I of France (a cousin of Catherine's mother), but he became heir to the throne when his older brother died in 1536. Francis died in 1547 and Henry acceded, with Catherine—who had become a prominent and highly esteemed figure in the court of her father-in-law—crowned queen consort in 1549. The couple's first child, Francis, was born in January 1544. They had waited a tension-filled ten years for Catherine to conceive the requisite heir to the throne, but once Francis was born her fertility was unleashed with a vengeance and between 1545 and 1556 she gave birth to nine more children, making a total of five boys and five girls. The last two, twin girls, nearly cost Catherine her life; and in 1559 an infection from a wound sustained in a jousting accident actually cost Henry his.

Throughout their entire marriage, Henry had had a mistress, a much older noblewoman named Diane de Poitiers, upon whom Henry had conferred all the political power that should have been Catherine's. Thus, when Henry died and Catherine's young and frail son Francis acceded, she was somewhat unprepared for the scheming political world into which she was suddenly thrown. France at that point was in a state of religious turbulence. The Protestant Reformation that began in Germany in 1517 had spread into France in the form of the Huguenots, a community that was rapidly gaining strength, and Francis found himself

> "A sinister Queen ... noted for her interest in the occult arts."
>
> *Gerald Gardner*, The Meaning of Witchcraft

Catherine de' Medici. *A stern portrayal of the queen consort of French king Henry II.*

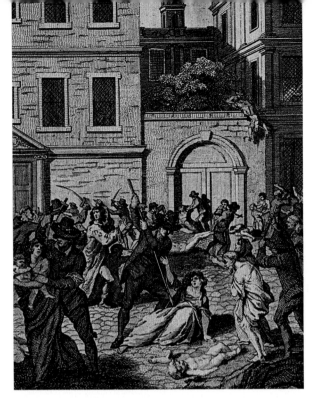

St Bartholomew's Day Massacre, August 24, 1572. *An engraving from Étienne Fessard, c.1780.*

dominated by the powerful and staunchly Catholic Guise family, who were engaged in persecuting the Huguenots to drive them out of the country. Huguenot retaliation was planned in what became known as the Conspiracy of Amboise, in which the young king was to be seized and overthrown. To Catherine's great relief, the coup d'état, in March 1560, failed; but Francis, always ailing, died later that year anyway, and his ten-year-old brother Charles became king with Catherine as regent.

THE WARS OF RELIGION

After the abortive coup, which led to the execution of all the conspirators except for one, Louis de Bourbon, a nervous Catherine attempted to mediate through the appointment of a humanist, Michel de L'Hospital, as chancellor. But while L'Hospital, supported by Catherine, advocated a policy of religious tolerance, the two sides remained unconvinced; and when a gathering of Huguenot worshipers was massacred at the instigation of the Guise family, the Protestant side felt they had no option but to take up arms, and signed a manifesto to that effect on April 12, 1562. Thus began the French Wars of Religion, characterized by horrific massacres of the Huguenots.

CATHERINE HATCHES A PLAN

Politically sound marriages have always been a feature of royal or influential families, and if ever there was desperate need for a strategic match in the French royal family, it was now. And Catherine, taking advantage of a momentary lull in hostilities, had an idea that she hoped would bring about a lasting peace and reconciliation between the two sides. She arranged the marriage of her youngest surviving daughter, Margaret, to Henry III of Navarre, a small kingdom sandwiched between France and Spain.

POISON CABINET

THE FRENCH SCHOOL OF POISONERS

By the second half of the sixteenth century, poisoning was so popular in France that those who used it with murderous intent were said to belong to the French school of poisoners, much as they might belong to a school of artists. Rumors of poisoning were as rife as the poisoners themselves, so it was not at all surprising that word should spread like wildfire that Catherine had poisoned Jeanne. And—since poisoning was almost an art form in itself—nor was it surprising that an exquisite pair of perfumed gloves should be declared the vehicle.

Henry was tailor-made for the job, having been baptized a Catholic but raised as a Protestant by his mother, Jeanne d'Albret. The wedding was to take place in Paris on August 18, 1572, and the only fly in the ointment from Catherine's point of view was that Jeanne was fiercely pro-Huguenot. She had become joint ruler of Navarre, with her second husband, Antoine de Bourbon (brother of the spared Amboise conspirator, Louis), in 1555, and when she converted to Calvinism on Christmas Day 1560, that branch of Protestantism was declared the kingdom's official religion, to the extent that Catholicism was banned outright. She lent practical support to the Huguenots throughout the French Wars of Religion and in 1570 negotiated a peace of sorts that allowed Huguenots to practice their religion in France.

SWEET GLOVES

Leather gloves, beautifully embellished with embroidery, tapestry, sequins, and lace, were a must-have fashion item in the sixteenth century. The only downside was that the leather tanning process at the time involved soaking the animal skin in human urine to remove the hair fibers. The urine was collected in "piss-pots" on street corners, a primitive form of restroom facility but one designed to serve the tanning industry rather than the comfort of the public. After this stage was complete, the skin was pounded with dung—often dog feces collected from the streets—or bated (soaked) in a solution of animal brains. This created a wonderfully smooth, supple leather with an utterly repulsive smell.

When Catherine arrived at the French court to marry Henry, she introduced an Italian custom that must have been more than welcome—the sweet glove, perfumed with a fragrant liquid derived from herbs, spices, and scented flowers.

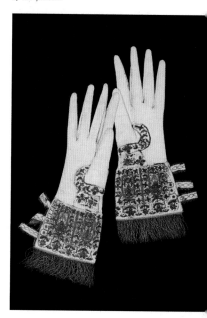

Sweet gloves. *A pair of gloves dating from the sixteenth century, in the style favored by fashionistas of the period.*

While Henry was the ideal match, Jeanne's religious leanings, and her doubts about the wisdom of the marriage, left something to be desired. But family is family, and it would be only good manners for Catherine to send a gift to her daughter's future mother-in-law—a pair of her very special gloves, a symbol of affection....

A SUDDEN DEATH

On June 9, 1572, just over two months before the nuptials between her son Henry and Catherine's daughter Margaret were to take place, Jeanne d'Albret died suddenly at the age of 43. Modern historians, unencumbered by the emotions felt by those under Jeanne's protection, believe the cause of death was nothing more sinister than tuberculosis; but the grieving Protestants of Navarre and France came to the inevitable conclusion that Jeanne's death, coming when it did, was not natural, and that she had been poisoned by none other than Catherine de' Medici, who was said to dabble in the occult and had even had horoscopes drawn up for her children by the celebrated seer Nostradamus. The consensus of opinion was that the vehicle for the (unidentified) poison had been a pair of the perfumed gloves for which Catherine was now so famous.

POSTSCRIPT

Jeanne d'Albret's death changed nothing. The wedding went ahead as planned, and was attended by many members of the Huguenot nobility. Less than a week later, just before dawn on August 24, St Bartholomew's Day, a massacre of Huguenots began in Paris, so brutal that the River Seine ran red with their blood. The following day, the massacre spread to the provinces. It transpired that Catherine de' Medici was behind the massacre, although her son, Charles IX, assumed responsibility, claiming that it had been triggered by a Huguenot plot against the crown.

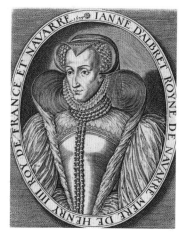

Jeanne d'Albret, queen of Navarre. *A depiction by the eighteenth-century French engraver Étienne Fessard.*

Henry of Navarre, on Charles IX's orders, reluctantly reverted to the Catholic faith, but later recanted, and when he was crowned king of France in 1589, there being no other heir, he had a battle on his hands since the French did not want a Protestant king. Finally, in 1593, Henry reverted to Catholicism for the last time, famously (or apocryphally) declaring that "Paris is well worth a mass." And his poor dead mother no doubt turned over in her grave.

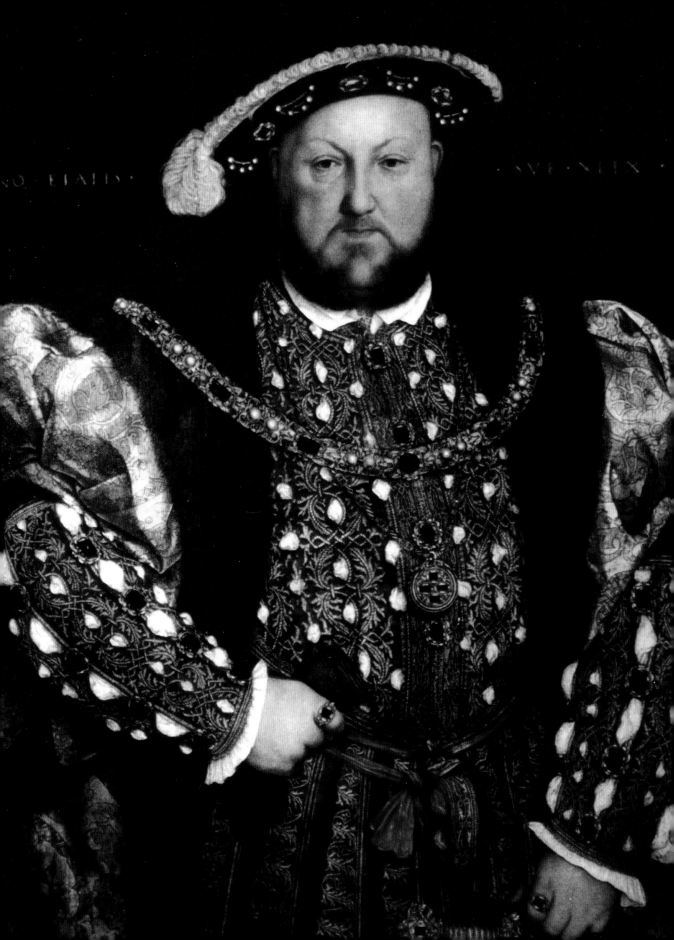

POISONING AT THE TUDOR COURT

England's flamboyant King Henry VIII is famous for many things, but none more so than his six wives. The fates of the first two, Catherine of Aragon and Anne Boleyn, were shaped by Henry's overwhelming desire to sire a male heir to the great Tudor dynasty. Anne Boleyn was keen to produce the heir herself—keen enough, perhaps, to poison a bishop who dared stand in her way.

O N AUGUST 22, 1485, the "Wars of the Roses," fought between the rival dynastic houses of Lancaster and York, came to an end when Henry Tudor seized the crown. England had lived through 30 unsettled years of bitter civil strife centered on who had the right to claim the throne, with one side gaining the upper hand for a time, only to lose it to the other. The story concluded, as so many of the best stories do, with a wedding.

A DYNASTY IS BORN

On January 18, 1486, the marriage of Henry Tudor, whose mother was of Lancastrian descent, and Elizabeth, daughter of the late Yorkist king Edward IV, took place in London's Westminster Abbey. The two rival factions were thus reconciled and united and England entered a new dynastic era: the Tudor period. Between 1486 and 1503, Henry and Elizabeth would have eight children; the first was a son and heir, Arthur, and the third was a "spare heir," Henry. On November 14, 1501, the lavish wedding of the young Arthur to Catherine of Aragon, daughter of the famous Spanish joint sovereigns Ferdinand and Isabella, took place in St Paul's Cathedral. Their union was to prove short-lived, however—just months later, on April 2, 1502, Arthur died. Henry became the new heir to the English throne and his father hastily negotiated a marriage treaty between Henry and his brother's widow in order to retain her dowry. A papal dispensation was sought and granted, on the (uncertain) grounds that the marriage of Arthur and Catherine had not been consummated.

Henry acceded on his father's death on April 21, 1509, and on June 11 he married Catherine. It ended an unsettled period for her, since she had for various reasons become less of a catch in the years since her betrothal to Henry in 1503; thus, by honoring the arrangement, her chivalrous new husband was her metaphorical knight (and literal king) in shining armor. Despite the unusual

King Henry VIII. *Not a man to mess with, as this 1540 portrait by Hans Holbein the Younger suggests.*

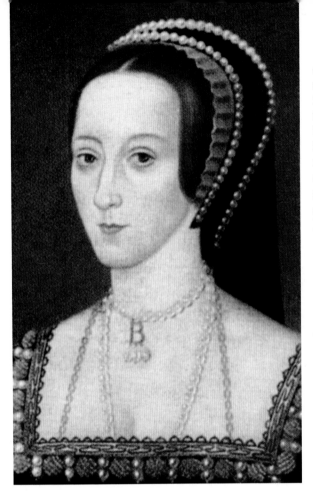

Anne Boleyn. *The object of Henry's affections is depicted here in a painting by an unknown artist.*

circumstances surrounding the union and a slight age difference—Henry was not yet 18 and Catherine 23 when they married—the couple muddled along together happily for many years, save for one thing: the matter of a male heir. Catherine was far from infertile—she conceived at least six times, but miscarried twice, and of three of the babies she delivered, one was a stillborn daughter and two sons died within weeks of their birth. The sixth baby survived; however, this was not the male heir Henry longed for, but a girl, Mary.

HENRY'S EYE WANDERS

Henry's issue was not exactly one of sexism, and indeed he recognized Mary as his official heir; but the memory of the dynastic struggle that was the Wars of the Roses was still fresh, the Tudor dynasty was still young and in need of strong guidance, and the previous attempt by a woman to rule England—the Empress Matilda in the twelfth century—had ended in anarchy and civil war. As precedents went, it was not an encouraging one. Catherine was clearly never going to produce a living son, and Henry began to wonder if it was time to rethink their relationship. Was he even married to her? Was the papal dispensation he had received in direct contradiction to the Bible? As the second son, Henry had originally been destined for the Church, and had studied theology. Could he use his knowledge of the Scriptures to get the marriage annulled, and start again with a new wife?

In fact, he already had a new wife in mind. Her name was Anne Boleyn, he was in love with her, and she was definitely not averse to becoming the new queen of England.

THE "GREAT MATTER"

Royal annulments were not uncommon, but when Henry sought one for himself, he immediately came up against an obstacle. The Holy Roman Emperor, Charles V, controlled the pope. He was also Catherine's nephew, so there was no chance that an annulment would be forthcoming from the pope without a fight. To add to the problem, Catherine had the support of Henry's courtiers, while Anne Boleyn was

---

THE 1531 ACTE FOR POYSONING

After the incident with Roose and the soup, Parliament passed a new bill, the Acte for Poysoning, which made it high treason to kill anyone with poison. Previously, it had been classified as a felony, for which the penalty was forfeiture of land and goods; high treason, however, incurred the death penalty. "Voluntary murderes [are] most highly to be detested and abhorred," asserted the terms of the act, "and specyally of all kyndes of murders poysonynge." And with those words, Roose was doomed.

unpopular. And at this point, Henry, who up until now had been a rather fine king and husband, became irrational to the point of obsession. He was convinced that he was right, and that the marriage was invalid and should be annulled, although he distanced himself from the whole thing by referring to it obliquely as the "great matter." Catherine, meanwhile, was equally convinced that *she* was right, and that the marriage was perfectly valid and should not be annulled.

BISHOP FISHER RAISES AN OBJECTION

The Tudor family had long had a close association with one Bishop Fisher, who had served as chaplain and confessor to Henry's paternal grandmother and as tutor to Henry himself. Fisher was deemed "the greatest Catholic theologian in Europe, without any rival" and Henry admired him greatly. When it came to the matter of the proposed divorce, however, Fisher predictably came down on the side of Catherine, declaring that the marriage was legal and could not be dissolved. He even took to writing books in support of her cause. Naturally, this did not please Henry—and it pleased Anne Boleyn even less. The subject of Henry asking the pope for dispensation to marry Anne (who categorically refused to become his mistress) had been mooted in August 1527 and by 1531 she was becoming a little irked at the lack of progress—so when on February 18 Bishop Fisher was served a bowl of soup that turned out to be laced with poison, rumors began to circulate that Anne had plotted to murder him, with the help of her equally ambitious family.

> "If a man shall take his brother's wife it is an unclean thing … they shall be childless." —*Leviticus*, XX, 21

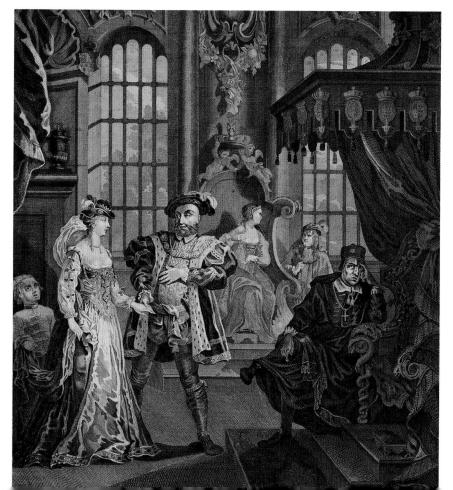

Love's young dream.
A portrayal of Henry courting Anne Boleyn, by an unknown engraver.

49

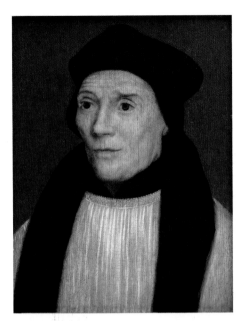

Bishop Fisher. *Painting by unknown artist. Fisher would not live to see England's transition to Protestantism.*

THE BISHOP ESCAPES DEATH

"Pottage" (soup) or "porrage" (gruel) was on the menu that day and, after drinking it, 17 members of Fisher's household who sampled it were "mortally enfeebled and poisoned." Fortunately, all but one—a man by the name of Bennett Curwen—survived. The bishop himself had no appetite that day and did not even taste the soup. There was another victim, however; the remains of the soup were given to a few poor villagers who called at the bishop's palace seeking alms, and one of them, the unfortunate Alice Tryppytt, also died. Was it food poisoning or a more sinister kind of poisoning?

When a problem with food arises, all eyes turn automatically to the person who produced it—in this case, one of the bishop's cooks, Richard Roose, who was promptly accused of adding "a certain venym or poyson" to the soup and charged with high treason. He is believed to have admitted to adding some powders to the soup but claimed that he thought it was only a purgative and that it was meant as a jest. The question of why he would in any case be so foolish as to attempt to murder his employer, the hand that fed him, was never raised, because on Henry's orders Roose was denied the chance to plead his case in the usual common-law trial.

"I COOKED THE COOK"

Richard Roose now had the unfortunate distinction of an entirely new method of execution being introduced specially for him, again on the orders of Henry, and passed by an act of Parliament. On April 15, 1531, less than two months after he served up his culinary disaster, Roose was taken to Smithfield, home of London's historic meat market and the site of many executions of heretics and political rebels, and boiled alive in a large cauldron, being "locked in a chain and pulled up and down with a gibbet at divers times until he was dead." Roose was not even allowed the benefit of a clergyman to ease his passing into the next world. A large and ghoulish crowd gathered to witness his demise, which took a full two hours. Only a few others were executed in this way before the method was deemed too severe even for the worst miscreant, and the law was repealed in 1547.

As for Henry, he never believed that his beloved Anne had anything to do with the affair, and is said to have enjoyed exclaiming gleefully: "I cooked the cook!"

> "He roared mighty loud, and divers women who were big with child did feel sick at the sight of what they saw."
>
> *An eyewitness to Roose's execution*

BISHOP FISHER IS EXECUTED

Bishop Fisher's feud with Henry over the divorce became ever more acrimonious. Henry decided there was only one solution to the great matter, and that was to break with the Church in Rome and have himself proclaimed Supreme Head of the new Protestant Church of England, thereby giving him the power to sanction his divorce from Catherine himself on the grounds that her marriage to Arthur *had* been consummated and that her marriage to Henry was therefore against God's law and invalid. In early January 1533, Anne Boleyn (having at last succumbed to Henry's charms) announced that she was pregnant, and Henry knew it was essential to marry her before the birth to ensure the child's legitimacy. The wedding took place soon after, on January 23, even though Henry's marriage to Catherine was not formally declared invalid until May 13.

In November 1534, the Succession to the Crown Act was passed, under which Henry's subjects—including the clergy—were required to take an oath to recognize Anne Boleyn as Henry's lawful wife and their children as legitimate heirs to the throne. Bishop Fisher refused to sign the oath, even after he was imprisoned, and on June 22, 1535, "his flesh clean wasted away and a very image of death," he was beheaded on Tower Hill—so called because of its proximity to the Tower of London, and another site of public executions, in this case those of high-profile traitors and criminals. As was the custom with traitors, his head was impaled on a pole on London Bridge, a warning to others who might feel inclined to disobey the monarch. He probably wished he'd had the soup....

Bishop Fisher's execution. *He was buried in the Church of St Peter ad Vincula on London's Tower Hill. Anne Boleyn joined him there the following year.*

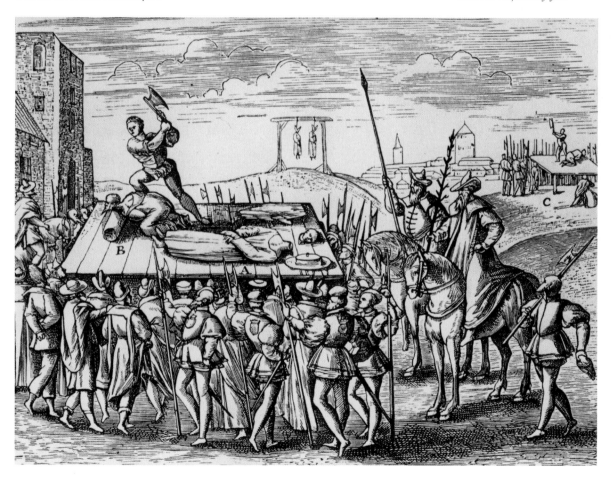

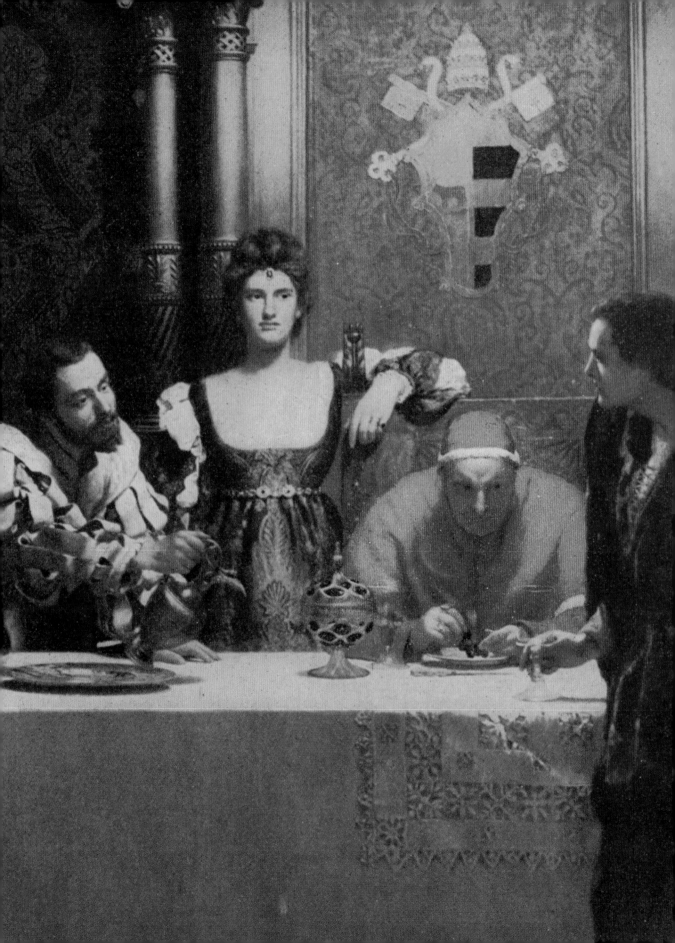

THE BORGIAS
A Family of Poisoned Poisoners?

The pope had been dead for less than a day. Yet mourners gingerly approaching the bier and peering into the dead man's face by the flickering candlelight had difficulty in suppressing their revulsion. His face was so swollen that he was unrecognizable— and it had turned completely black. It was put about that he had died of poison; further gossip said that he had accidentally drunk doctored wine intended for his dinner host. Could it be true that Rodrigo de Borgia, whose name in modern times has become synonymous with poison, had actually died by his own hand?

R ODRIGO HAD BEEN BORN 73 years earlier into a wealthy family in Xàtiva, in eastern Spain. The family name, Borja, would be changed to Borgia, judged less foreign-sounding for an Italian audience. Rodrigo's uncle Alfonso was already bishop of Valencia; he encouraged the boy to study law and when, in 1455, Alfonso became Pope Callixtus III, he promptly made the 24-year-old Rodrigo a cardinal.

THE SPANISH INTERLOPER

The Borgias were incomers to the fiercely Italian Holy City, and none of the prominent Italian families who surrounded them ever let them forget it. Nevertheless, and despite the fact that his uncle and mentor died in 1458 after a papacy lasting under four years, Rodrigo's standing increased steadily; he was smart, cynical, and a naturally astute politician.

The form of the papacy in the fifteenth and early sixteenth centuries would not be recognizable today. The church wielded secular as well as spiritual power; popes and cardinals were expected to be adept politically and socially. They often attracted nothing stronger than formally expressed disapproval for living very unholy lives—many accrued huge fortunes by selling favors within the church, kept numerous mistresses, and lived like kings in extremely luxurious courts.

Such circumstances suited Rodrigo Borgia very well. By shrewdly managing the favors at his disposal, he increased his wealth until he was one of the richest of the cardinals, with palaces, art, and a household to match. Famous for his

The Borgia family. A *nineteenth-century rendering of the villainous trio, Cesare and Lucrezia Borgia and Alexander VI. Cesare offers poisoned wine, while Lucrezia looks on, implacable—and Rodrigo is clearly plotting his next outrage.*

The Borgias   **53**

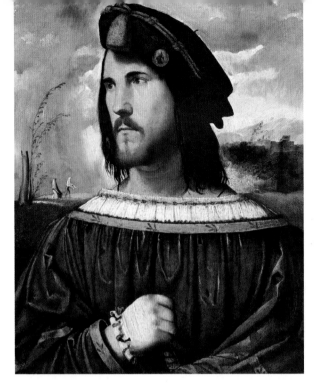

Cesare Borgia. *Painted by Altobello Melone, this portrait justifies his reputation as the handsomest man in Europe. He even modeled for the likeness of Christ in the murals Rodrigo commissioned for the Borgia apartments.*

"Never presume that I will not act on my worst instincts." —*Cesare Borgia*

admiration of beauty, he took as his long-term mistress Vannozza dei Cattanei, an aristocrat who was well known for both her looks and her savvy business sense (she ran a number of successful lodging houses in Rome). She bore him four children, two of whom, Cesare and Lucrezia, would become just as notorious as their father. Although his intimate relationship with Vannozza would end in around 1480—long before he became pope—Rodrigo must have cared for her. While many churchmen disowned their children, he acknowledged and supported his, and provided for Vannozza throughout his life. (She would outlive him by 15 years, eventually dying at the grand old age of 76.)

A POWERFUL FAMILY

In 1492, Rodrigo Borgia was elected pope, taking the name Alexander VI. No one doubted that he had done it by bribing many of his fellow cardinals, but after all, he was not the first Borgia to become pope, and even those who disliked him admired his intelligence and subtlety.

His two middle children with Vannozza seemed to have proved the most interesting to him. The oldest of the four, Juan, was murdered in 1497; the youngest, Gioffre, made a successful marriage to the daughter of the king of Naples. Cesare and Lucrezia, though, had inherited both their father's brains and their mother's looks. From childhood, Lucrezia was admired for her beauty. She had hazel eyes, waves of silky blond hair, and an elegant profile—the last a quality particularly admired by fifteenth-century portraitists. At the age of just eight she was sent to live with a cousin of her father's, who taught her all the fashionable accomplishments—dancing, singing, drawing, and conversation. By the time she was 11, an engagement had been arranged for her; at 12, she posed for the artist Il Pinturicchio, who depicted her as a luminous St Catherine in the frescoes he was painting in Rodrigo's apartments. At the age of 13, her original engagement by now broken, since when her father became pope he could afford to be even more ambitious for her, she was married off to Giovanni Sforza, a nephew of the powerful Duke of Milan.

Cesare was educated for the Church and, already created archbishop of Valencia, when his father became pope Cesare was made a cardinal aged just 18. He was as good-looking as his sister, and as clever, self-interested, and political as his father. The Renaissance author Niccolò Machiavelli spends a great many words on Cesare Borgia in *The Prince*, his classic study of the attainment and management of power, although even Machiavelli might have had difficulties with the depth of Cesare's ruthless streak.

And ruthless both Rodrigo and Cesare undoubtedly were. Their enemies were dealt with quickly and without sentiment, and many ended up dead. Rodrigo's chief ambition was to pull the principal Italian city-states, constantly in conflict, back under the control of the papacy, and it was with this in mind that in 1496 he put his son at the head of the papal army. Cesare was still only 20 years old.

LUCREZIA: SAINT OR SINNER?

The lurid gossip that surrounded Lucrezia during her lifetime still clings to her name over 500 years later. But was she really the depraved monster Romans loved to talk about? Almost certainly not. Whereas there is plenty of evidence for the darker deeds of her father and brother, Lucrezia's main crime seems to have been to agree to act as their matrimonial pawn, and in that age, an aristocratic woman would have had little choice. Her first marriage was annulled after her husband allied with the French—who were at the time invading Italy—against Cesare (and it was probably an aggrieved Giovanni Sforza who first started the rumors of her incestuous relationships). After a decent interval spent in a convent, she married Alfonso of Aragon in a match that was once more arranged by her father and brother. The young couple were fond of one another, but their union, in turn, became less advantageous a couple of years later when Cesare swapped sides and formed an alliance with Louis XII of France, to whom Aragon stood in opposition. Alfonso was first threatened with poison ("Don't forget," Cesare is said to have taunted him after they shared a meal, "what didn't happen at lunch may still happen at dinner...") and then was murdered, almost certainly on Cesare's orders. Lucrezia, who seems to have been both shocked and in mourning, agreed to a third marriage shortly after, this time to Alfonso d'Este, heir of the Duke of Ferrara. She was still just 21 years old.

In Ferrara, away from her family, she seems to have thrived and, finally, to have been happy. She gradually won over her father-in-law, a grim elderly widower, and managed her relationship with her husband while simultaneously conducting a number of courtly love affairs. Her refinement, liveliness, and beauty were all appreciated and the Ferrara court came to love her. She was sincerely mourned when she died in 1519, having outlived both Rodrigo and Cesare. It was recorded that Alfonso wept copiously as he knelt by her bier.

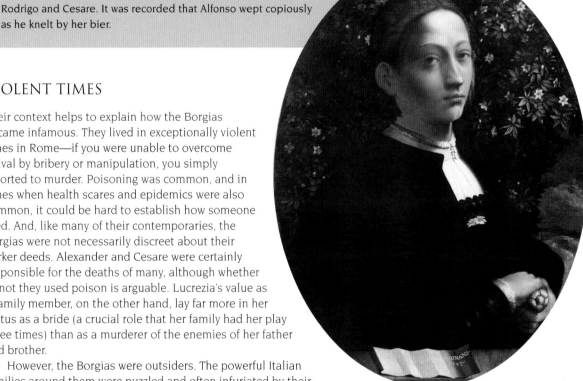

Lucrezia Borgia. *A disputed portrait of Lucrezia, purportedly by the Renaissance master Dosso Dossi. The ambiguous expression and hooded eyes fit her allegedly scheming personality, which would become the stuff of legend*

VIOLENT TIMES

Their context helps to explain how the Borgias became infamous. They lived in exceptionally violent times in Rome—if you were unable to overcome a rival by bribery or manipulation, you simply resorted to murder. Poisoning was common, and in times when health scares and epidemics were also common, it could be hard to establish how someone died. And, like many of their contemporaries, the Borgias were not necessarily discreet about their darker deeds. Alexander and Cesare were certainly responsible for the deaths of many, although whether or not they used poison is arguable. Lucrezia's value as a family member, on the other hand, lay far more in her status as a bride (a crucial role that her family had her play three times) than as a murderer of the enemies of her father and brother.

However, the Borgias were outsiders. The powerful Italian families around them were puzzled and often infuriated by their

POISON CABINET

Cantarella, the mythical poison of the Borgias, acquired a fearsome reputation among their rivals. It was said to have a slightly sweet taste, making it easy to disguise in wine or sweetmeats. It was entirely undetectable and could kill in minutes, days, or weeks, depending on the dosage.

Did cantarella really exist? No sample was ever obtained nor any analysis made, but contemporaries alleged that it was a powerful mixture of arsenic, copper, and phosphorus—with the extra revolting detail that it was "prepared in the decaying carcass of a hog," the entrails of which were then pressed, and the liquid thus extracted was dried to a powder before being deemed ready for use.

success. It stood to reason that they must have some special means, and from quite early on in Rodrigo's career he was accused of using poison to dispose of unwanted rivals. Rumor became accepted fact—Lucrezia was alleged to use her beauty to entrance her victims—and then to prick them with a needle on a special ring with a compartment full of poison. Cesare, too, was said to be a master of the art of poison, able to calculate a dose of the family's unique recipe, a poison called "cantarella," to the point where he could predict a death to the minute. Never mind that Cesare's rivals were often discovered to have been stabbed or strangled—poison made for a much better story. These Spanish foreigners were unnaturally close, too, Romans muttered—Lucrezia and Cesare were obviously lovers, and Rodrigo's affection for his daughter was evidence of a much more sinful relationship.

THE FINAL BANQUET

In August 1503, the pope and his son were invited to a dinner at the home of Adriano Castellesi, a powerful cardinal. August was not a popular month for dining out in Renaissance Rome, as the summer air in the crowded city was foul, and the "miasmas" that came up from the Tiber were held to be unhealthy, but the Borgias went anyway. The story that circulated later was that they had sent some cantarella-laced wine ahead of them as a gift, but had accidentally drunk it when it was served, instead of leaving it untouched as they had intended. Whatever the truth of the matter, by the following day both Borgias and Cardinal Castellesi were violently ill. The cardinal and Cesare would survive (despite the treatment prescribed by Cesare's doctors, which saw him suspended for an hour in a barrel full of iced water), but Rodrigo died. The reign of the second Borgia pope was over.

"Her whole being radiates good humor and joy beyond words."

Nicolo Cagnolo of Parma, diarist, of Lucrezia

Johann Burchard, papal master of ceremonies at the Vatican, left a gruesome account of what happened directly after Rodrigo's death. Cesare sent some of his men to guard the pope's apartments, where the cardinals appointed to the task were making an inventory of the vast number of valuables, and they promptly ransacked many items. In the meantime, Rodrigo's body was carried, first to the Sistine Chapel, and then to the basilica. Menaced by armed soldiers, the attendants fled, leaving the body of the pope unwatched. By 4pm that afternoon, when Burchard saw the corpse again, he reported: "Its face had changed to the color of mulberry or the blackest cloth and it was covered in blue-black spots … the appearance of the face then was far more horrifying than anything that had ever been seen or reported before."

Priests were too frightened to attend the body of the unloved pope. He was dumped in the nearby Church of Santa Maria della Febbre, where carpenters and porters jammed his swollen corpse into a coffin several sizes too small, swearing and joking as they did so. It was too short for his miter, which was crammed in alongside him.

Did Alexander VI die from poison, inadvertently administered by his own hand? Modern historians believed that the real cause of death was an acute attack of malaria—one of the reasons that Romans disliked humid summer dining. But the frightening state of the corpse, which in less than a day became bloated and black, still leaves the question open for discussion.

And what happened to Cesare? The new pope, Julius II, was a sworn enemy of the Borgias, and Cesare was swiftly placed under arrest and subsequently returned to Spain, where he was imprisoned. On his escape, he hired himself out to the king of Navarre and, while laying siege to the castle of one of the king's enemies, was ambushed and killed. More than 25 stab wounds were counted on his body. He is buried in Viana, Spain, where he fell, under the inscription: "Here, in a scant piece of earth lies he whom all the world feared." The age of the Borgias was truly over.

> "Too much mercy allows disorders to go on, from which spring killings or depredations."
>
> Niccolò Machiavelli, The Prince

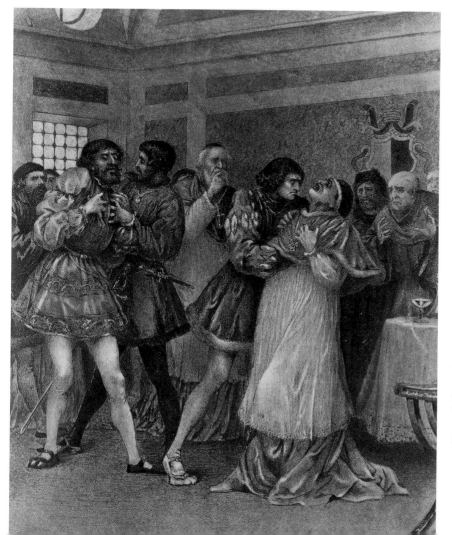

Death at the banquet. *Plenty of artistic license has been taken in this engraving showing the poisoning of the Borgias. Clutching their throats, seemingly already poisoned, Cesare and Alexander are apparently being helped on their way by a pair of menacing assassins.*

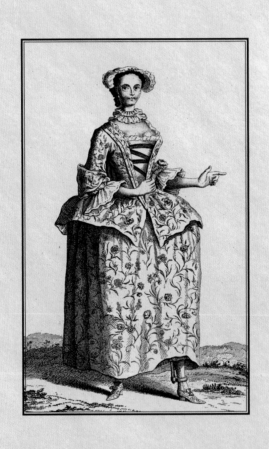

CHAPTER THREE

MURDER IN THE 17th & 18th CENTURIES

In the 17th and 18th centuries, using poison as a means of dispatching someone in the way was the preserve of the well-to-do middle and upper classes. Dispensing with the need for blunt instruments and bloodshed, it even had a whiff of sophistication about it. Mary Blandy, English gentlewoman, never let standards slip. Even when incarcerated pending trial for poisoning her father, she was depicted taking tea with a companion in dainty fashion, despite sporting leg irons beneath her capacious gown. More than one member of the French aristocracy took to poison with gusto, including the Marquise de Brinvilliers whose exploits had the courtiers of Louis XIV looking over their shoulders nervously. And the infamous Marquis de Sade poisoned—albeit accidentally—two young women with Spanish fly, an aphrodisiac but lethal in too generous a quantity. An instance of taking the pursuit of the arts of love to the extreme.

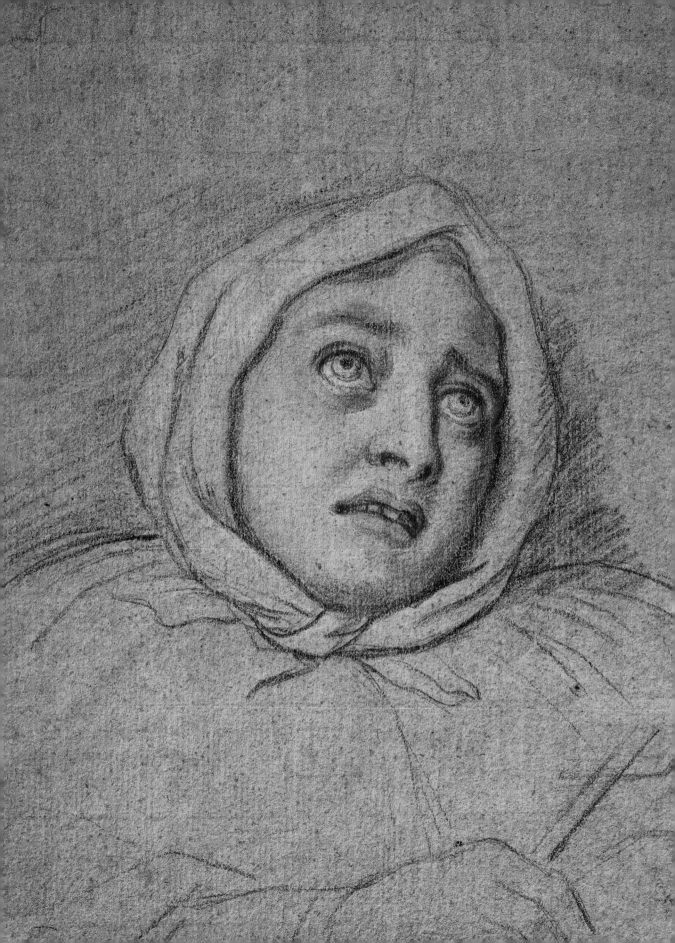

THE AFFAIR OF THE POISONS

In 1676, a French noblewoman, the Marquise de Brinvilliers, was beheaded for poisoning assorted members of her family. The matter did not end there, however—it sparked an investigation into other courtiers of Louis XIV, the Sun King, including his beautiful (but insecure) official mistress. The tribunal would be forever known as "The Affair of the Poisons."

LOUIS XIV ACCEDED to the French throne on May 14, 1643, when he was just five years old. From the very start, he was destined to be the center of his own universe—his birth had ended a 23-year wait for an heir, and he was immediately hailed as "Louis the God-given." It is not surprising, then, that he chose the sun as his personal emblem, or that his courtiers revolved around him like the planets in the solar system. He certainly did not expect the people in his court to be troublesome.

THE MARQUISE DE BRINVILLIERS

Marie-Madeleine-Marguérite d'Aubray was born around 1630, the daughter of a civil lieutenant of Paris. She married Antoine Gobelin de Brinvilliers, an army officer, in 1651, but in 1659 he made the mistake of introducing her to his dashing rogue of a best friend, Jean-Baptiste Godin de Sainte-Croix, who promptly became her lover. The marquise's outraged father, Antoine Dreux d'Aubray, intervened to end the scandalous and widely publicized affair, and in 1663 Sainte-Croix found himself detained in the Bastille, the French state prison. He was not amused, but it appeared that luck was on his side. During his incarceration he made the acquaintance of an Italian fellow prisoner, known as Exili, who was a renowned chemist and poisoner. Exili shared his knowledge of toxins with Sainte-Croix, and when he was released a year later, the handsome roué plotted with the Marquise de Brinvilliers to vent his feelings with some well-aimed poisoning.

The pair did not rush to execute their plan, though, but spent two years testing the poisons. Sainte-Croix obtained them and when the marquise visited the poor and the sick, she distributed alms, sympathy, and a dose of something

> "One only has to look at her to see she was scheming something."—Louis XIV's *sister-in-law,*
>
> *speaking of the Marquise de Montespan*

Marie-Madeleine d'Aubray. *A sketch of the Marquise de Brinvilliers on her way to the scaffold, attributed to the French court artist Charles Le Brun.*

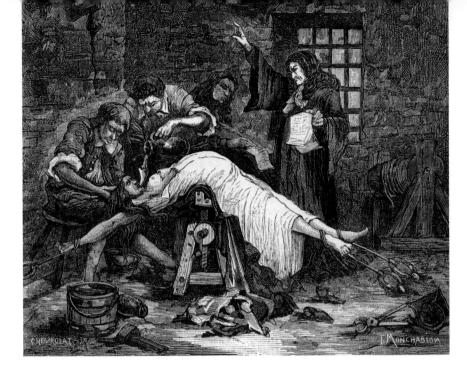

Water torture. *The "ordinary"
and "extraordinary" questions—
water torture combined with being
stretched either on a rack or over
a wheel—was so agonizing that
a full confession was almost
guaranteed, whether the victim
was guilty or not.*

toxic so she could note the effects and identify the poison least likely to be detected (they are thought to have decided on a recipe concocted by another Italian poisoner, Giulia Tofana, see page 63). The marquise thus dispatched some 50 victims before even making a start on the intended targets. The original plan had been to poison the marquise's father, Antoine Dreux d'Aubray, who had so ruthlessly had Sainte-Croix jailed. But Sainte-Croix was now facing financial ruin, so the marquise's two brothers and sisters were doomed to die too, in order for her to inherit the entire family fortune. The marquise was also keen to poison her husband, but it seems Sainte-Croix balked at the prospect of marrying his murderous mistress, and spared the life of his former friend.

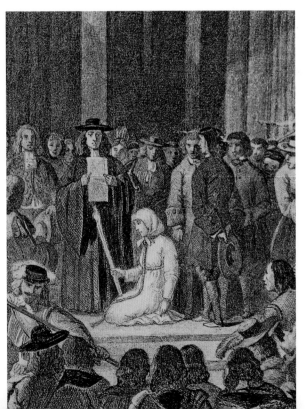

The trial of the Marquise de
Brinvilliers. *This set aristocratic
nerves jangling throughout Paris
and ultimately led to many
startling revelations.*

DE BRINVILLIERS DETECTED

Despite their best efforts, it did not work out as the pair had planned. In February 1666, they poisoned the marquise's father. In 1670, they poisoned her two brothers. But on July 31, 1672, before they poisoned the marquise's sister, the last link in the chain, Sainte-Croix himself, died suddenly, possibly in the midst of an experiment. And to make matters worse, he left evidence incriminating his partner in crime and their coconspirator, a servant nicknamed "La Chaussée," who had aided and abetted in the murder of the marquise's brothers. Unfortunately for the Marquise de Brinvilliers, the evidence fell into the hands of the Paris gendarmerie—the police.

La Chaussée was arrested, tortured into a full confession, and executed on a Catherine wheel, a singularly unpleasant device to which the offender's intertwined limbs were lashed and then beaten until they broke. The marquise, meanwhile, fled the country, only to end up being lured to a convent in Liège by a representative of the French authorities disguised as a priest. Her attempt to commit suicide was thwarted, and she was returned to Paris, where on July 16, 1676, having been subjected to water torture until she confessed, she was beheaded and her body cremated. But she had left lingering in the air a very significant observation, made during her interrogation: "Half the people of quality are involved in this sort of thing, and I could ruin them if I were to talk." She could not have condemned those "people of quality" more effectively if she *had* talked.

LA VOISIN

The Marquise de Brinvilliers' trial and revelation left King Louis and his courtiers feeling decidedly on edge, wondering constantly if someone had designs on their life. They began to look askance at mysterious deaths, wondering just how "mysterious" they really were. Louis is even said to have gone to the extreme of having a servant test his food to make sure it was safe before he tucked in himself (servants, unlike monarchs, were expendable). And there wasn't only poison to be feared—there were black masses, spells, aphrodisiacs…

One woman in particular was very popular among those wishing for a little occult assistance in their dubious endeavors, Catherine Monvoisin, known simply as "La Voisin." At the time of the Affair of the Poisons, she was in her mid-30s, and had many talents at her disposal—she was a midwife (and abortionist), a clairvoyant and fortune-teller, and skilled at performing black masses and dishing out potions and poisons. She cleverly transformed herself into a brand; when it came to carrying out darks deeds, who could resist consulting a woman dressed in a flowing crimson velvet robe embroidered with mystical symbols in gold thread? The fact that she lived in the Paris slums did not deter her aristocratic clientele, and perhaps even added to her mystique.

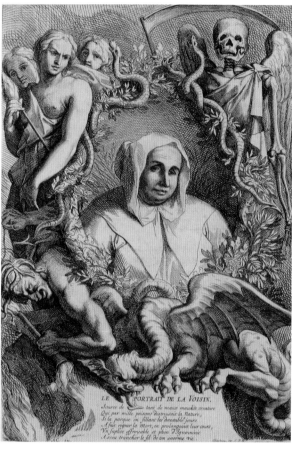

La Voisin. *A contemporary line engraving of the aristocracy's favorite sorceress, surrounded by sinister images of black magic and death.*

POISON CABINET
AQUA TOFANA

The poison Aqua Tofana was the deadliest of its era. It was colorless, odorless, tasteless, and foolproof—it is thought that it was used to poison more than 600 male victims. It was based on arsenic, belladonna, and lead, and a mere four drops could relieve a woman of an unwanted husband (or father and/or brothers). The genius of its inventor, Giulia Tofana, lay in her trick of secreting the poison in a bottle disguised as a healing ointment, so no one would guess its lethal contents.

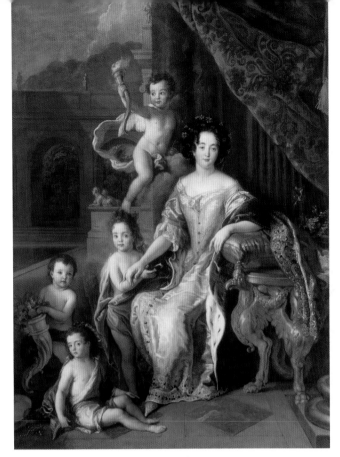

Madame de Montespan.
Official mistress of Louix XIV,
Montespan gave birth to seven of
the king's children, as well as two
sired by her husband.

THE MARQUISE DE MONTESPAN

The Sun King was unaware that he had been subjected to La Voisin's dark art long before the Brinvilliers trial. In 1660, he had married his cousin, the Spanish Infanta. In common with most royal marriages, it was a political alliance and, as was also common, the king soon acquired a "maîtresse-en-titre" (official mistress), Mademoiselle de la Vallière. The position of official mistress was much sought after, and in 1667 Louis fell under the spell (literally, as it turned out) of a very alluring usurper, the Marquise de Montespan, a member of the queen's household, who had enlisted the aid of the obliging La Voisin. The marquise—also commonly referred to as Madame de Montespan—had attempted fruitlessly for a year to divert the king's attention from Mlle de la Vallière ("She tries hard, but I am not interested," declared Louis), but once she had administered La Voisin's love potion of bats, toads, the blood of deceased infants, ground-up human bones, and a winning combination of herbs, Louis was lost. The mesmerizing marquise held the king's attention for a decade, fending off attempts by younger women to take her place.

LOUIS ORDERS AN INQUISITION

In 1677, a Parisian woman named Magdelaine de La Grange, whose range of shady skills was similar to those of La Voisin, was arrested and charged with poisoning her lover, and like the Marquise de Brinvilliers, she hinted at crimes committed by prominent courtiers. The king was sufficiently unnerved by this latest revelation to order Gabriel La Reynie, chief of the Paris gendarmerie, to investigate. The zealous officer rounded up all the city's known alchemists and fortune-tellers and one by one, under torture, forced them to disclose the names of their clients.

In 1679, Louis set up an extraordinary court, known as a *chambre ardente*, to try the accused, both those who provided the means to commit the crimes and the criminals themselves. The trial lasted just over a year, during which time well over 400 people were interrogated. Thirty-four were sentenced to death; others were exiled, and many imprisoned.

> **CHAMBRE ARDENTE**
> The *chambre ardente* ("burning tribunal") was established in 1535 by Jean, Cardinal of Lorraine, an advisor to King Francis I of France, to try heretics found guilty by the inquisitorial tribunal. Francis's son Henry II made fulsome use of the court in his bid to expel the Protestant Huguenot community from the country. The origins of the tribunal's name are unclear, but carry sinister connotations of heretics burning at the stake.

DE MONTESPAN TURNS MOODY

Among the courtiers who were implicated in the case was the king's own official mistress, Madame de Montespan. Louis, who was starting to find his mistress's unpredictable temper a little tiresome, had taken a new lover with whom he was besotted, promptly giving her the title Duchesse de la Fontanges. The marquise was not pleased. She had spent many years as the "epicenter of the court, its pleasures and its fortunes," as Louis' godson, the chronicler Saint-Simon, observed, and she did not appreciate being displaced in favor of a 17-year-old said to be as stupid as she was beautiful. The marquise's response, it emerged, had been to visit La Voisin and ask her to poison Louis. La Voisin plotted to deliver a petition, coated in poison, into the king's hands. She duly arrived at court on March 5, 1679, armed with her quirky murder weapon, only to discover that Louis was not granting audiences that day. It was to be her only attempt on his life—she was arrested, found guilty of witchcraft, and on February 22, 1680, she was burned at the stake.

DE MONTESPAN DETECTED

When the king's mistress, the Duchesse de la Fontanges, died suddenly in 1681, La Reynie suspected foul play. La Voisin's daughter alleged that Madame de Montespan had not only purchased aphrodisiacs from La Voisin but had taken part, naked, in satanic rituals to perpetuate the king's passion for her, and had asked La Voisin to poison the duchess. La Voisin's daughter was not the only one to have mentioned the marquise's name, and La Reynie's interest was piqued. But in 1682, before La Reynie could act upon his suspicions, Louis unexpectedly brought the tribunal to a close and abolished the *chambre ardente*. He signed *lettres de cachet*, which authorized suspects to be imprisoned without trial or right of appeal, and he ordered all the evidence and witness statements that had been gathered throughout the tribunal to be sealed and secured in a locked chest, along with all the court papers. The case had been closed. Literally.

DE MONTESPAN GETS OFF SCOT-FREE

If La Reynie was unhappy about the abrupt termination of his investigation, he was not prepared to raise his head above the parapet and risk incurring the wrath of the king. As for Madame de Montespan, no proof was ever found of any of the crimes she was alleged to have committed; but although she continued to live at the royal court, her days as Louis' official mistress were over and she was replaced by Madame de Maintenon—a humiliating outcome, as Louis married his new mistress on the death of his wife in 1683. Madame de Montespan retired from the court in 1691 and ended her days in a Parisian convent. She was fortunate—but for Louis stepping in to close down the tribunal, her death would almost certainly have been significantly gruesome.

> "If these crimes are hidden, what other strange and unknown things will befall…"
>
> *Gabriel La Reynie*

Gabriel La Reynie. *Chief of the Paris gendarmerie, La Reynie led the investigation into the Affair of the Poisons.*

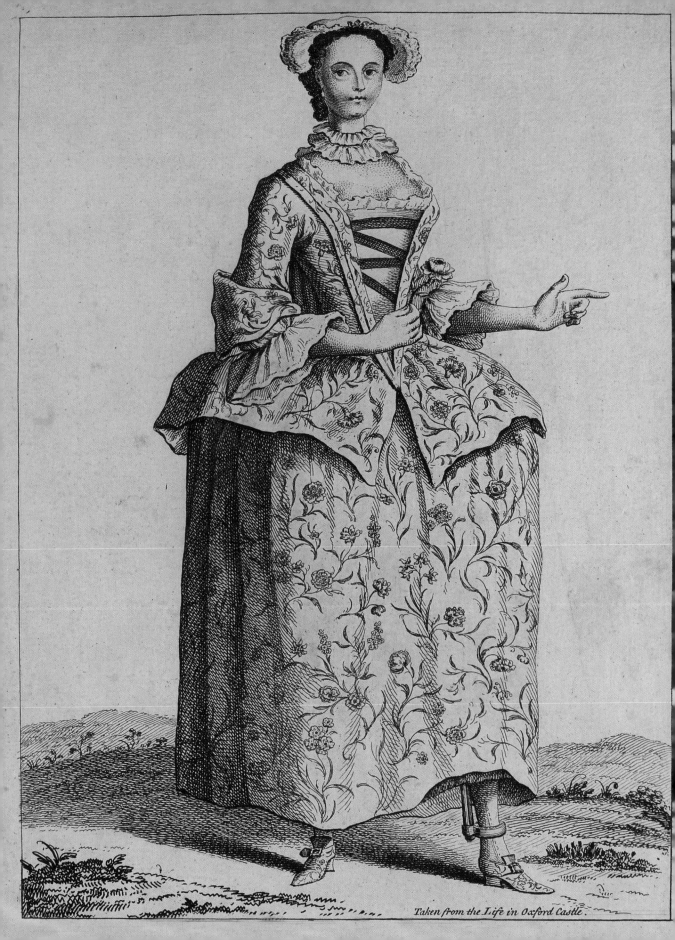

Taken from the Life in Oxford Castle.

MARY BLANDY
The Respectable Parricide

Was she a cold-blooded murderer, or simply a fool for love? The dark story of Mary Blandy has divided opinions for more than two and a half centuries. Whatever the truth of the case, her trial remains notable for being the very first in which science was used to determine the victim's likely cause of death—it saw the birth of forensics.

MARY WAS the only child of Francis Blandy, a town clerk and attorney, and his wife Anne. The family lived in middle-class comfort in Henley-on-Thames in Oxfordshire, England, and Mary was said by those who knew her to have been a bright and attractive child. Although her looks were marred by an early attack of smallpox that left her with bad scarring, she grew into an elegant and accomplished girl. She was judged clever, charming, and "amiable," and her socially ambitious father had high hopes that she would find an appropriately agreeable and wealthy husband.

But the years passed and no one that Francis Blandy deemed suitable came calling. Mary was in her mid-20s—and by eighteenth-century standards, well and truly on the shelf—when, in 1746, her father hit on the idea of adding a dowry to her appeal. He made it known that the lucky man who married her would be rewarded with £10,000 (worth around 200 times as much or over 2 million dollars today) by his rich new father-in-law. Suddenly, there was no shortage of gentlemen eager to court Mary, but the aspirational Francis had high standards and rejected all applicants. Some weren't ambitious enough, others didn't make the grade financially, while still others didn't rank high enough socially to be partnered with his precious only child.

One man, however, was not prepared to be so easily dismissed. When Mary first met William Henry Cranstoun he seemed a safe enough acquaintance. He was the nephew of General Mark Kerr, a friend of her father. Henry doesn't seem to have been a heartbreaker. He, too, had been badly marked by smallpox; in addition, he was short with "clumsy" legs (particularly unlucky at a time when a well-turned calf displayed in fine hose was considered an important feature of a gentleman), his eyes were small, and his conversation—in contrast to Mary's—was inelegant. Nevertheless, he was a captain in the army and, music to the ears of the snobbish Francis Blandy, he was also the fifth son of Lord Cranstoun, a Scottish peer.

> "I gave it to my poor father innocent of the effects it afterwards produced."
>
> *Extract from* Miss. Mary Blandy's Own Account, *1751*

Mary Blandy. A *contemporary engraving of Mary, "taken from life at Oxford Castle," where she stayed while on trial. The artist has given her an elegant and fashionable appearance, slightly marred by the leg irons fixed around her dainty ankles.*

THE BIGAMOUS SUITOR

Whether or not Mary was initially reluctant, something about Cranstoun won her round. Perhaps she was becoming desperate to be married to someone of whom her family approved, perhaps Cranstoun had some elusive charm that was not recorded in contemporary accounts. Whatever the truth of it, the couple were soon walking out together with the full approval of her parents, with a marriage expected shortly. And during Cranstoun's frequent absences over the border, Mary sent him affectionate letters, addressed to "Dear Willy."

The Blandys' happy plans were abruptly ruined by General Kerr. On hearing news of the engagement, he brusquely informed Mr Blandy that Cranstoun already had a wife and a child in Scotland. William told an altogether different story. He owned that the lady in question, Anne Murray, had been his mistress and that they had had a child, but denied that he had ever intended to marry her. By way of reassurance he added that the case was currently being heard in the Scottish courts and it would shortly be confirmed that he was neither married nor promised to anyone else. In fact, it appears that he *was* legally married, despite his denials, but in any event, his argument

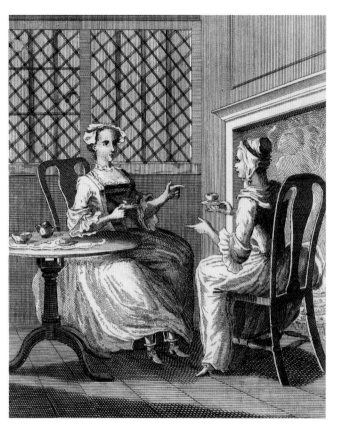

Entertaining in prison. A *genteel Mary takes tea with a female visitor. Only the bars at the windows and the irons on her legs reveal that she is not in her own parlor.*

did nothing to help his case with Mary's father. Francis Blandy was furious; Mary was forbidden to see Cranstoun again. The wedding—bigamous or not—was off.

However, Mary did not forget Cranstoun. The couple stayed in touch, and continued to meet clandestinely. Mrs Blandy was sympathetic to their cause; she appears, inexplicably, to have remained partial to Cranstoun, but in the autumn of 1749 she fell ill and died shortly afterward. Mary was left alone with her unresolved affair, apparently still in thrall to her untrustworthy suitor, yet forbidden by her father to meet or communicate with him.

Cranstoun, although he had lost an advocate in Mrs Blandy, had not forgotten the £10,000. The miserable business dragged on; he continued to write to Mary and to press his suit, and to meet with her whenever it could be managed, but neither knew how to overcome her father's objections. Late in 1750, Cranstoun proposed a possible solution. He knew, he said, a wise woman who specialized in potions and who had suggested she supply one of her mixtures which Mary could hide in her father's food. Cranstoun told Mary that the effect of this "friendship" or "forgiveness" powder would be to soften Francis's attitude toward him, enabling them finally to marry.

THE FORGIVENESS POWDER

Just how credulous was Mary? Could she really have believed him? By this time she had good reason to know that Cranstoun was a liar; at some point, he had actually confessed to her that he was married, still stressing that he hoped to be released before long. Nevertheless, early in 1751, he sent her the supposed forgiveness powder. He took the trouble to disguise it, sending it with a packet of semiprecious pebbles—there was a vogue for polishing them and using them in jewelry at the time—and the packet was labeled "the powder to clean the pebbles with." Mary began to administer it to her father, slipping small quantities into his food and drink. Francis quickly became unwell, vomiting after meals, complaining of cramps and stomach pains. He had previously suffered from kidney stones, and later Mary would claim that she had thought the symptoms marked the return of his complaint. Even when his teeth began to fall out and he became unable to take anything but gruel, she continued to dose him. The powder was actually arsenic.

Some members of the household were becoming suspicious. On one occasion a maid finished a bowl of gruel that had been intended for Francis and was promptly taken ill herself, with terrible stomach cramps and vomiting. On August 6, Mr Norton, the local apothecary, was called in to advise on the case. (An apothecary's visit was one step down from a visit from a doctor; the latter was usually called in only for very serious illness.) Mary appeared to be dancing attendance on her father, but he was getting sicker and sicker, often complaining of the sensation of a "fireball" in his stomach. Just a few days after the apothecary's visit, it was evident that Francis Blandy was dying. Servants later claimed that he had directly accused Mary of poisoning him and, perhaps frightened by this, she called Dr Anthony Addington to attend him on August 10.

The possibility that Francis was being poisoned seems by this point to have been openly discussed in the household. A grainy residue was noticed at the bottom of one of Blandy's interminable bowls of gruel. Susan Gunnell, one of the servants who would later give key evidence at Mary's trial, scraped it out, folded it into a paper, and later gave it to Dr Addington, and the doctor told Mary quite frankly that she might be suspected of poisoning her father. It may have been this that panicked her into making a fire to burn Cranstoun's letters and what remained of the powder he had sent. She was interrupted in the process by another of the servants who pulled the remains of a packet out from the flames and set it to one side.

POISON CABINET

ARSENIC

"White" arsenic (that is, arsenic burned to combine with oxygen, then crystallized as a lethal powder) was one of the commonest poisons available in the eighteenth century. It was used to whiten lace, to kill vermin, as a component of face powder and other cosmetics, and even appeared in minute quantities in various medicines. Its effects when taken in larger quantities are cumulative and agonizing: a fiery, pricking sensation in the victim's tongue and throat, a difficulty in swallowing, quickly followed by unbearable burning sensations in the stomach and continuous vomiting. Mr Blandy's end would not have been a comfortable one.

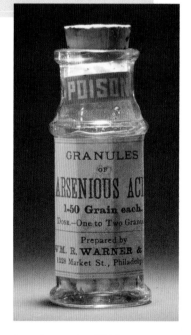

Arsenic granules. *Widely available in the eighteenth century, Mary claimed that she thought the powdered arsenic was a potion that would soften her father's attitude toward her lover.*

"I TESTED THE POWDERS"

Poisoning, whether accidental or by design, was far from uncommon in the eighteenth and nineteenth centuries. Numerous toxic substances were used for cleaning, getting rid of vermin, or even, in smaller quantities, as medicine, and there were few accurate tests to identify them. The case of Mary Blandy stands out because Anthony Addington, the doctor who attended her father in his last agonies, attempted to test the substances found in Francis's food and in the packet Mary had tried to burn against some classic tests for arsenic. He found that, when burned, the powder smelled of garlic, and when mixed in a glass of water, it left a film on the water's surface while a gritty substance sank to the bottom—both ways in which arsenic was known to behave. By today's standards the tests were very primitive indeed, but they gave weight to the suspicions of Mary and added a modern, scientific gloss to the evidence against her.

Mary Blandy   **69**

On August 14, 1751, after several visits from Dr Addington, Francis Blandy died. By this time, gossip had become widespread locally. At the doctor's suggestion, Mary was confined to the house. When the day after her father's death she managed to break out (claiming she merely wanted to take a walk and breathe the fresh air), she was pursued by a crowd of locals, shouting and harassing her, and was forced to take shelter with a friend at a nearby inn.

> "The crime with which the prisoner stands charged is of the most heinous nature and blackest dye."
>
> *Judge Legge, addressing the jury at Mary's trial*

ARREST AND TRIAL

On August 17, Mary Blandy was formally arrested, charged with the crime of parricide, and removed to Oxford Castle, where she was held for some months while her trial was prepared. She was far from idle during her imprisonment. She gave interviews to interested parties, she contributed to articles and broadsheets about her case, and she published *Miss. Mary Blandy's Own Account*, which portrayed her as a loving daughter and the innocent dupe of the villainous Cranstoun. She had become notorious; engravings of her taking tea with a lady companion, looking attractive and demure despite being hobbled by leg irons, were printed by pamphleteers and sold to the public in hundreds.

Meanwhile, what became of Cranstoun? On hearing of Mary's arrest, he abandoned her completely and fled to France, disappearing from the story, although it is known that he died in November 1752, in Flanders, without ever returning to England.

Oxford Castle. Despite its forbidding appearance, Mary's accommodation here was comparatively comfortable; she had a large room with its own fireplace and warm blankets to see her through the winter.

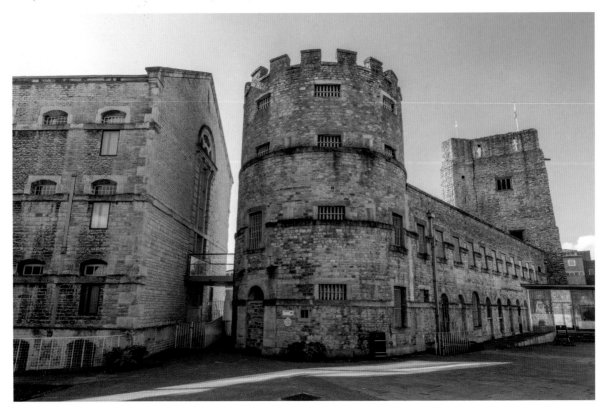

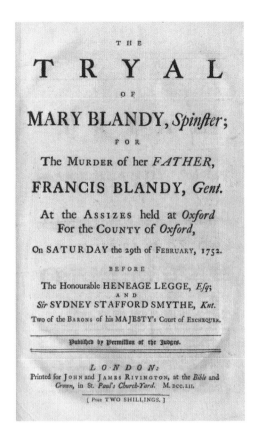

THE

TRYAL

OF

MARY BLANDY, *Spinster*;

FOR

The MURDER of her *FATHER*,

FRANCIS BLANDY, *Gent.*

At the ASSIZES held at *Oxford*
For the COUNTY of *Oxford*,

On SATURDAY the 29th of FEBRUARY, 1752.

BEFORE

The Honourable HENEAGE LEGGE, *Esq;*
AND
Sir SYDNEY STAFFORD SMYTHE, *Knt.*
Two of the BARONS of his MAJESTY's Court of EXCHEQUER.

Published by Permission of the Judges.

L O N D O N:
Printed for JOHN and JAMES RIVINGTON, at the *Bible* and
Crown, in St. *Paul's Church-Yard.* M.DCC.LII.

[*Price* TWO SHILLINGS.]

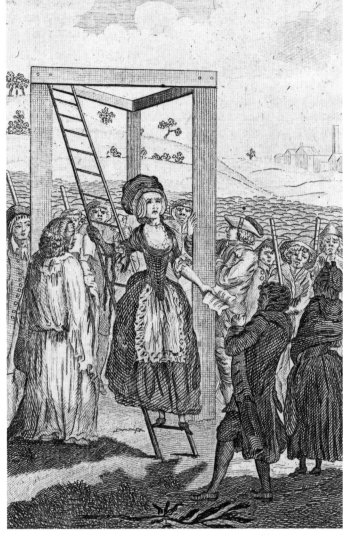

Mary's execution. *This rough engraving shows her addressing a large crowd from the ladder of a very improvised-looking scaffold. The trial—and verdict—had been widely discussed in pamphlets distributed all over Britain.*

Mary's trial took place on March 3, 1752. The opinions of onlookers remained divided. Some of the servants said that Mary had been an unkind daughter, while others claimed she had been both dutiful and affectionate. Mary freely admitted that she had given the arsenic to her father, but maintained, variously, either that she had believed Cranstoun's story or that she wanted to appear to believe it to keep his affection. She was adamant that she had believed the powder to be harmless. Despite the damning evidence, some who saw her on the witness stand believed her when she said, "I really thought the powder an innocent, inoffensive thing, and I gave it to procure his love." For the prosecution, Dr Addington's novel evidence about testing the powder for arsenic added some scientific gravity to the trial. After 11 hours of evidence had been heard, the jury took just 15 minutes to find Mary guilty.

Mary Blandy was hanged at Oxford on April 6. She maintained her innocence to the very end, and went to the gallows in a tasteful black silk gown with matching black ribbons. Her final thought on the scaffold seems to have been to guard her modesty: "For the sake of decency, gentlemen," she appealed to her executioners, "don't hang me high." Whether or not she had murdered her father deliberately, she still didn't want the hoi polloi looking up her skirt.

There is a final irony to the story. When Francis Blandy's will was read, it emerged that his entire estate consisted of just under £4,000. Mary's £10,000 "dowry" had been a figment of her father's imagination. Had Cranstoun actually married Mary, he would have been a disappointed man.

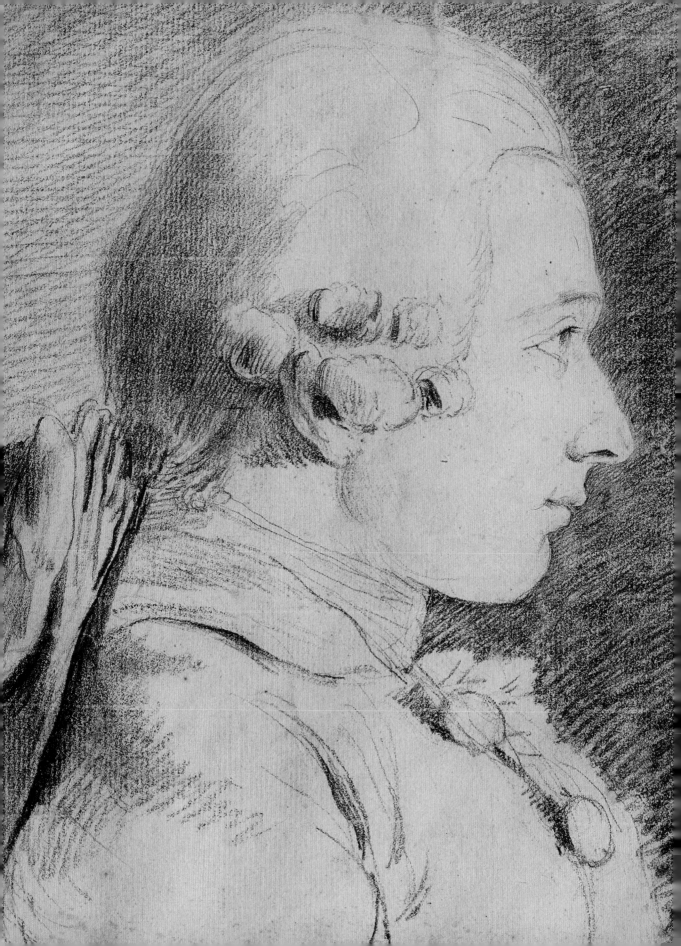

MARQUIS DE SADE
The Toxic Orgy

He was already famous as a libertine but the Marquis de Sade's orgy, held in Marseilles on June 27, 1772, had repercussions severe enough to affect the rest of his life. In the short term, it would lead to imprisonment, although this was already hardly a novelty for the 32-year-old aristocrat. Well over two centuries later the true facts, obscured almost immediately by scandal, gossip, and—in the case of some of the more prurient commentators, at least—wishful thinking, will probably never be known.

POISONER

Donatien Alphonse François, Marquis de Sade
Born: June 2, 1740, Paris, France
Died: December 2, 1814, Charenton, France
Motive: Accidental; poison taken as an aphrodisiac
Poison: Cantharidin (a chemical more commonly known as "Spanish fly")
Number of victims: Exact number unknown

D E SADE HAD BEEN BORN into an aristocratic family in Paris. His mother, Marie-Eléonore de Maillé de Carman, was lady-in-waiting to the Princesse de Condé; his father was a lieutenant-general for a number of provinces and had served as ambassador to the court of Russia and minister plenipotentiary to the elector of Cologne. Young Donatien, born at the Condé court, was educated from the age of six by his uncle, the Abbé de Sade, at the latter's estate in Saumane-de-Vaucluse in the Auvergne region of central France. When the boy turned ten, he was sent back to Paris to spend a few years at a Jesuit school before being accepted at the army training academy at Versailles.

By 1756, when the Seven Years' War broke out between France and Prussia, he was serving as a second lieutenant in the King's Light Infantry and in 1757 he moved to the Carabiniers, where, aged just 17, he became a standard bearer. His army career ended with the war, and does not seem to have hindered young de Sade's romantic or sexual education. By his early 20s, he was already consorting with prostitutes and boasting of the philosophical freedom his debauchery gave him. Aristocratic French society in the second half of the eighteenth century was far from prudish. Provided that you followed some basic rules and conducted your affairs in private, you could largely behave as you pleased. Unfortunately, the young marquis had a tendency toward exhibitionism.

> "Either kill me or take me as I am, because I'll be damned if I ever change."
>
> *The marquis writing to his wife, November 1783*

Donatien Alphonse François, Marquis de Sade. *The marquis aged 20, in an elegant pencil drawing made by Charles-Amédée-Philippe van Loo. It is the only portrait known to have been taken from life.*

MARRIAGE AND THE FIRST SCANDALS

Early in 1763, he found himself in a dilemma. His family had engaged him to Renée-Pélagie de Montreuil, an heiress from a rich and influential family; meanwhile, he had engaged himself to a second girl, Laure de Lauris, who came from an aristocratic family in Provence, with whom he genuinely appears to have been in love. De Lauris seems eventually to have rejected him; at any rate, that summer he married Mlle de Montreuil, who, reputedly plain, quiet, and devoutly Catholic, was to serve as his devoted wife for decades.

> "If anyone so much as whips a cat in this province, the gossips all say, 'It's Monsieur de Sade who did it.'"
>
> *The marquis complaining of his notoriety in 1775*

Marriage failed to turn the marquis respectable. He rented a clandestine apartment on the Rue Mouffetard in Paris, a private place for him to practice his increasingly disreputable habits. Shortly after his wedding, he met a pair of prostitutes there for a modest orgy; unfortunately, he made the mistake of defiling a crucifix in the course of it. Blasphemy was taken rather more seriously than debauchery, and when the prostitutes complained to the police, de Sade found himself imprisoned in the Château de Vincennes just outside Paris. Rather touchingly, he was keen that his new wife should not discover the nature of his crime, letting it be known that he was locked up because of his debts. He was back home by the beginning of 1764, and continued to combine marriage with private adventures of his own.

In 1767, Renée-Pélagie gave birth to the first of the couple's three children, Louis-Marie. Less than a year later, de Sade was the focus of a major and widely publicized scandal. A woman called Rose Keller who, according to different accounts, was either a beggar or a prostitute, had met de Sade on Easter Sunday, April 3, 1768, on the Place des Victoires in Paris. She negotiated to go to his apartment—either to clean it or for sex, depending on whose story you believed. When she went into the bedroom, he strapped her to a bed, whipped her viciously,

The Château de Lacoste.
The de Sade family's ancestral home in Provence, and a favorite refuge for the marquis when he had taken things too far.

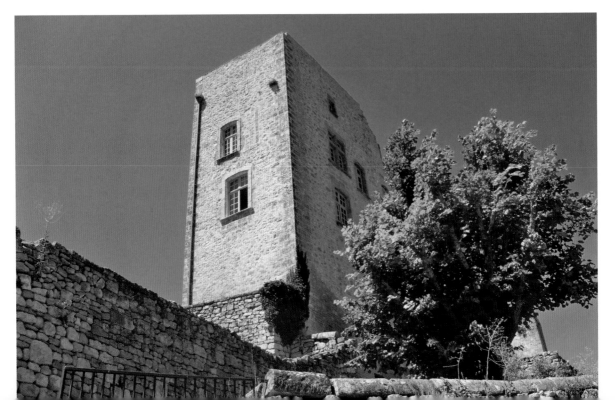

and then dripped hot candle wax into her cuts. When he had satisfied himself, he untied her, allowed her to wash, and offered her ointment for her wounds. She had feared for her life during the encounter, however, and went straight to the authorities. By June, the marquis was back in prison, where he remained for almost a year. When he was released, he retired to the Château de Lacoste, one of the ancestral de Sade properties in the Luberon district of Provence. He took with him his wife and her younger sister, with whom he was already having an affair.

From this point on, the authorities kept a much closer eye on de Sade. Licentious behavior in the French aristocracy was nothing new, but there was an extreme quality about his activities that worried them, and the unsurprising hostility of his wife's parents ensured that he remained under surveillance.

THE MARSEILLES AFFAIR

From late 1769, life for de Sade seems to have quietened down for a while. But the peace was shattered when, accompanied by his manservant, Latour (and, as the press would titillatingly report, "his partner in sodomy"), de Sade made a trip to Marseilles in June 1772. Officially, the purpose of the visit was to collect some money he was owed, but it seemed a pity to leave the city without indulging some of his other tastes. Latour was instructed to hire an apartment and some young prostitutes so that the marquis could enjoy an orgy before returning home to the country.

Latour duly made arrangements with a popular local madam, Mariette Borelly. When de Sade arrived, three young prostitutes were waiting for him, and he and Latour had an enjoyable afternoon and evening, organizing and partaking in every imaginable sexual combination, no doubt including bondage and flagellation. In between their exertions, the girls were given refreshments, among them chocolate pastilles, offered in a crystal box. Probably unused to such elegance, they devoured the treats, but the bonbons had been laced with Spanish fly, a well-known aphrodisiac and, incidentally, a poison. By the following day, the women were enduring terrible stomach pains. Weak and vomiting, they went to the police, complaining that de Sade had made an attempt on their lives. An order for his arrest went out on charges of poisoning—and sodomy.

Had he meant to poison them? Almost certainly not—he probably simply intended to add a final fillip to his orgy. But the rumor mill was soon in full flow; he had poisoned the girls on purpose, the gossips said, and, they went on, several had died. The numbers involved rose, too—from a handful of people, those reported to have attended the party went from ten to twenty to fifty....

A flavor of the local outrage can be felt in a quote from one local commentator: "The most modest women," he salivated, "were unable to restrain themselves." Although quite what a modest woman would have been doing attending a party held by a nobleman by now notorious throughout France, if not throughout Europe, is open to question.

POISON CABINET

Cantharidin, known more commonly as "Spanish fly," was the offending substance the delinquent marquis offered his guests. It is extracted from meloid or blister beetles (hence the poison's informal name). It was used by the Roman empress Livia to induce people to commit sexual indiscretions. The beetles use its irritant effect to guard their eggs and deter predators, but its reputation as an aphrodisiac came from the powerful itching it causes, particularly in the mucous surfaces of the genitals.

In women, "the itch" was believed to create a powerful lust satisfiable only by constant sex; in men, the irritation of the urethra led to an erection which could last for hours or even, after a heavy dose, days. Taken in excess, it can have a range of effects, from intense stomach pain and palpitations to kidney failure and serious heart and breathing problems, followed, if the victim is unlucky, first by a coma, and, ultimately, death. While there is no evidence that anyone at de Sade's orgy died, the reputation of Spanish fly as a dangerous indulgence was well deserved.

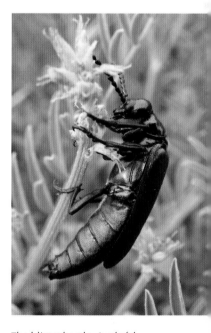

The blister beetle. *A colorful insect whose excretions—used by the beetle to repel predators—can be put to much less innocent purposes when they fall into the wrong hands.*

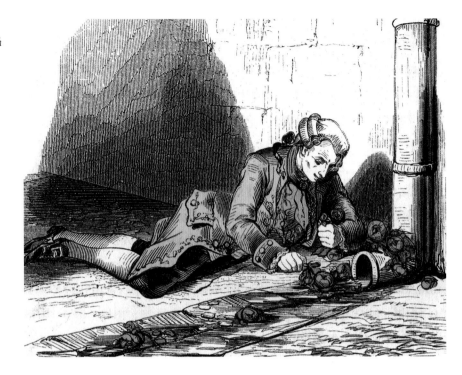

The marquis imprisoned. *In this engraving he is toying with roses, emptied from a vase; in reality, however, he spent his prison days writing busily. His draft of* The 120 Days of Sodom, *for example, was over 250,000 words long.*

THE MARQUIS CONFINED

By the time the news was out, de Sade was back home in the Luberon. He and Latour were sentenced to death in their absence by the thoroughly overexcited authorities (and their effigies hanged in public), and spent some time in Italy evading arrest. When he was finally captured, powerful friends interceded on his behalf and he was simply shut up in the Château de Miolans in Savoy from where, in 1774, he would escape out of a window. Soon he was back at Lacoste, living with his long-suffering wife, several young servant girls, and a male secretary.

The local girls were probably his undoing this time. When it became clear that the sort of services they were providing did not include housework, their parents complained, and the weary authorities once again sentenced de Sade. When he was returned to prison in February 1777, this time to the Château de Vincennes, it was for the long term. In 1784, he was transferred to the Bastille, then, in 1789, sent to the insane asylum at Charenton, southeast of Paris, an unusually humane institution for its time, where his opinions were allowed free rein and he was able to write. He spent much of his incarceration writing— not only his famously obscene novels and stories, but also endless lengthy letters to his wife. Many of these survive, and the picture they paint is rather unexpected. They are filled with minor moans and complaints: the caps that Renée has bought for him are too small; the fruit she sent in was unripe; not enough is being done to keep him comfortable. Far from reinforcing his image as the wickedest man alive, in his letters, the marquis comes across as a querulous fusspot.

"Let the traces of my grave disappear from the face of the earth, as I flatter myself that my memory will be effaced from the mind of men."

Extract from de Sade's will, written in 1806

THE REVOLUTION AND AFTER

De Sade was finally freed in April 1790. His wife left him at around this time, although after enduring his extramarital exploits for so long, quite what the final straw can have been is hard to imagine. The revolutionary government, however, felt no distaste for de Sade. He set his hand to writing revolutionary pamphlets and was soon appointed secretary of the Les Piques section, an area of Paris incorporating the Place Vendôme. But at the end of 1793 he was accused of *modérantisme*—moderatism, a new crime in revolutionary law—and only narrowly escaped the guillotine. He was released, once more, in 1794.

By this time, the marquis was out of money and no longer a figure of influence. He had a new partner, a young actress and single mother, Marie-Constance Quesnet, but lack of funds forced him to sell the family home at Lacoste in 1796. He was still trying to earn a living from his writing—he wrote plays as well as pornography—but had limited success.

The rise of Napoleon saw de Sade's final fall from grace. The new middle-class code of values found de Sade genuinely shocking, and although his novels *Justine* and *Juliette* had been published anonymously, he was soon identified, and in 1801 he was tracked down while visiting his publisher, arrested, and imprisoned without trial. His family sensibly had him declared insane in 1803, allowing him to be moved back to Charenton, where he spent his final 11 years in a largely benign regime, unrepentant, untamed—and for the most part cheerful—writing, casting the inmates in his plays, and seducing the 13-year-old daughter of one of the prison warders. He finally died on December 2, 1814, still notorious, though no longer the svelte wrongdoer of his youth; he suffered from rheumatism and had become immensely fat.

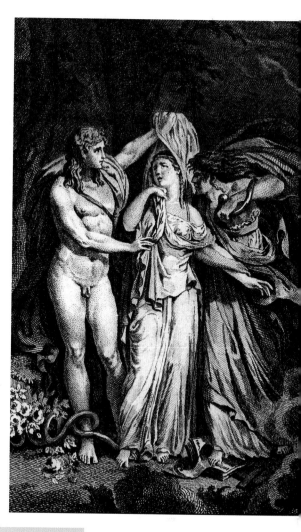

Engraved illustration for de Sade's Justine. *Pornography given a "classical" gloss. In the text, the virtuous and put-upon Justine does not remain clothed for very long.*

THE GREAT PHILOSOPHER

De Sade's writings can be forgotten in the rollicking saga of his life. But he wrote incessantly, and, given that he spent almost three decades of his life locked up, he had plenty of time to do so.

His first work, T*he 120 Days of Sodom*, was written in the Bastille on a single roll of paper almost 39 feet (12 meters) long. Today's readers might find it too repetitive to be effective as pornography and not coherent enough to be judged as philosophy (the category in which its author would certainly have placed it). If it was written to shock, though, it certainly succeeded. De Sade's other best-known works, *Justine* (1791) and *Juliette* (1797), were also tales of innocence defiled in many imaginative ways. They were banned from publication shortly after his death, and did not become widely available until the 1960s. The books are now erotic classics.

Was de Sade a great thinker? He certainly thought so, and subsequent admirers included the poet Guillaume Apollinaire and many of the surrealists, including Man Ray and Salvador Dali. They saw a freedom in his thinking, a moral darkness, that goes far beyond mere pornography.

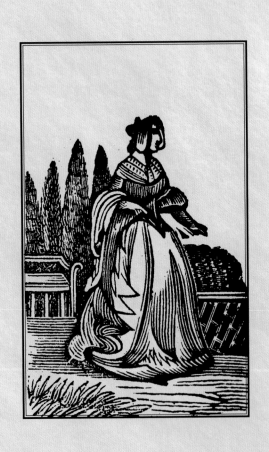

CHAPTER FOUR

THE GOLDEN AGE
OF POISONING

For poison to have a golden age is a dubious accolade, but "doing away" with an associate or family member for amorous or financial gain has proved too much of a temptation for many over the years. Administering the poison invariably involved stealthy and furtive measures, with the poison of choice often being concealed in some tempting foodstuff, such as a slice of cake. Or worse, the poisoner would administer the dose to the trusting and unwitting victim as "medicine," disguising their lethal intent with apparent concern and kindness. Arsenic, to some extent the epitome of poisons and legally present in the dye used in many perfectly innocent items from toys to wallpaper, became a firm favorite in the Victorian era. But when poison began to be used on an industrial scale in warfare, it paved the way for mass civilian poisonings to come.

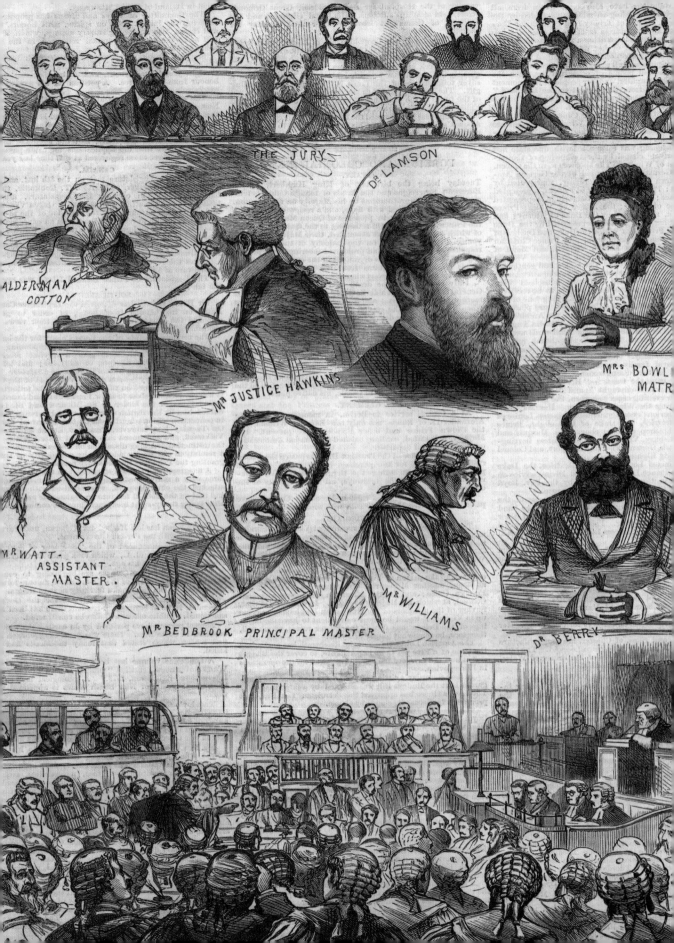

THE JURY

ALDERMAN COTTON

Mr JUSTICE HAWKINS

Dr LAMSON

Mrs BOWL MATR

Mr WATT ASSISTANT MASTER.

Mr BEDBROOK PRINCIPAL MASTER

Mr WILLIAMS

Dr BERERY

GEORGE HENRY LAMSON
The Sleight of Hand Murder

Dr George Henry Lamson was the picture of Victorian respectability, living with his wife and baby daughter in an equally respectable English seaside resort. But Dr Lamson had a dark secret, an addiction, and to feed this addiction he needed money. He knew where he could get it, and all it would take was a traditional fruit cake with one extra ingredient....

POISONER

George Henry Lamson
Born: September 8, 1852, New York City, USA
Died: April 28, 1882, Wandsworth, London, England
Motive: Financial gain
Poison: Aconite
Number of victims: 1

G EORGE HENRY LAMSON'S life started out full of promise. He was born on September 8, 1852, in New York City, to the Reverend William Orme Lamson and his wife, Julia. The family later moved to England, where George attended medical school and qualified as a surgeon. So far, so good.

LAMSON GOES TO WAR

In July 1870, war broke out between France and Prussia. The Prussian side quickly proved its superiority; the French emperor, Napoleon III was captured and France was declared a republic. Prussian forces besieged the French capital, Paris, intent on starving the citizens into submission; however, the French, ever resourceful where gastronomy is concerned, hastily invented "siege cuisine" and, far from starving, enjoyed such delicacies as horse soup, dog cutlets, and fricassee of rats and mice. When they ran out of livestock, pets, and rodents, they ate animals from the zoo. The Parisians might not have been happy, but they were not dying of starvation in huge numbers, and the Prussians, losing patience, gave up waiting for the surrender and brought in heavy siege guns. Paris is said to have sustained more damage in the bombardment than in any other conflict, before or since.

And here we find our hero, Lamson, serving as a medical officer with the French Ambulance Corps and doing an excellent job. When the war ended, Lamson became the proud wearer of the French Legion of Honor, the country's highest order of merit. It was the first of many such awards he would earn in Eastern Europe over the next few years, and he rounded off his success by cutting death rates in his ambulances by 30 percent while serving with the Romanian Army during the Russo-Turkish War of 1877–78. Thus it was a triumphant young man who arrived in the English coastal resort of Bournemouth in 1878, armed with glowing testimonials from armies all over Europe, to take up a position as a general practitioner.

Trial by jury. The trial of Dr George Henry Lamson, illustrating the accused, the trial lawyers, and the star witnesses who exposed the ulterior motive behind Lamson's gift of cake.

THE LURE OF MORPHINE

As a medical officer in war-torn countries, Lamson was more than familiar with injecting his injured and dying patients with morphia (morphine) to relieve their pain. Morphine, an opiate found naturally in plants, had been isolated by a German pharmacist, Friedrich Sertürner, in the early nineteenth century. It was marketed commercially from 1827, and when the hypodermic syringe was invented soon after, it became an easy-to-administer analgesic. But it is also addictive, and the authors of Lamson's glowing testimonials were unaware that he himself had become addicted.

Lamson could not have made a better choice than Bournemouth for his new home in England. Unusually, in a country littered with towns and cities many hundreds of years old, Bournemouth had only been founded in 1810. Marketed as a health resort, it quickly grew in size and popularity, and among its affluent visitors were many who were also addicted to morphine, which was freely dispensed from a pharmacy conveniently close to Lamson's house.

KEEPING UP APPEARANCES

A doctor, however dark his secrets, must present a respectable face to the world, and Lamson worked hard at it. In addition to his general practice, he received a commission as a medical officer in the Bournemouth Artillery Volunteers and, most significantly, he got married. His wife, Kate John, was one of five children, but one sister had died, leaving her with one sister and two brothers. When their parents died, each child received an inheritance, payable when they came of age or were married, whichever was the sooner. Since the Married Women's Property Act was still in the future, Mrs Lamson's inheritance passed to her husband, who promptly spent it. When Kate's brother Herbert died the year after her marriage, she inherited more money, which Lamson also spent.

By 1881, things were looking ugly. Lamson now had a baby daughter, a failing medical practice, and a string of very embarrassing debts. The bank stopped honoring his checks, his house was sold, and he was reduced to pawning his worldly goods. This was not the image a decorated war hero wanted the world to see. He had become very creative in his excuses for not repaying his debts. Now it was time to get creative where replenishing his coffers was concerned.

> "The dark angel of death had got him in a relentless clutch."
>
> *From the evidence for the prosecution*

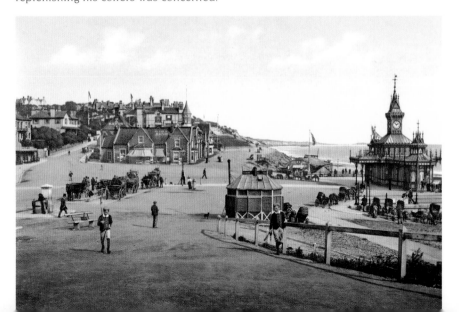

Bournemouth in the 1870s. A *Victorian coastal resort located on England's south coast. Outwardly the essence of respectability, the town was a magnet for morphine addicts.*

THE YOUNG PERCY

Kate's surviving brother, Percy, had curvature of the spine and was paralyzed in his legs, although he was otherwise healthy. He was at school in Wimbledon, southwest of London, where his fellow pupils willingly helped to look after him. It was not the perfect life, because Percy could not participate in the sporting activities enjoyed by the other boys, but within its limitations it was certainly pleasant.

Percy was the only legatee in his family who had yet to claim his inheritance. At the height of Lamson's troubles, Percy was still two years away from his coming of age, and marriage in the interim seemed unlikely. Were he to die, his two surviving sisters would each receive half of his considerable inheritance. Lamson wanted that money.

In the early evening of December 3, 1881, Lamson visited Percy at his school. Both Percy and the school's headmaster, Mr Bedbrook, observed that Lamson had become pale and thin, although they were of course unaware of the reason. Mr Bedbrook offered Lamson a glass of sherry, and Lamson, rather bizarrely, asked for some sugar to add to it. A bemused Mr Bedbrook sent for a bowl of sugar. Lamson then produced a Dundee cake—a spicy Scottish fruit cake— already sliced. He handed a slice to Percy, containing a raisin heavily laced with the poison aconite, while both he and Mr Bedbrook also ate a slice (unpoisoned). He now produced a new innovation he had discovered on a recent visit to America, a gelatin capsule. He made a great show of filling one with sugar from the bowl and inviting Percy to swallow it, to demonstrate to Mr Bedbrook its ease and usefulness for administering medicine to his pupils. Percy obliged.

PERCY MEETS HIS DEATH

As soon as Percy gulped down the capsule Lamson departed, with indecent haste, to catch a train—he was en route to Paris. As he was walking Lamson to the door, Mr Bedbrook commented on Percy's deteriorating physical condition, and Lamson expressed the opinion that Percy's days were numbered. And how right he was— after several hours of violent convulsions, vomiting black fluid, and complaining of intense pain in his stomach, that his skin felt "drawn up," and that his throat was closing, Percy died. Ironically, he was given morphia to ease his suffering.

A FAILED SLEIGHT OF HAND

A postmortem suggested the cause of death was "the administration of some poison." Meanwhile, a highly suspicious Mr Bedbrook informed the police. On his return from Paris, Lamson was arrested, and here everything went wrong. Lamson presumed that suspicion would fall upon the sugar-laden capsule—of which he could, of course, claim to be entirely innocent, having sampled the sugar in his sherry. No one, he reasoned, would give a second thought to the cake—but the vexatious Mr Bedbrook did. When it was discovered that Lamson had recently purchased aconite from a London pharmacy, his options for denying all knowledge ran out. The jury at his trial quickly found him guilty. He was hanged on April 28, 1882, his short and sorrowful life a salutary lesson in the perils of addiction.

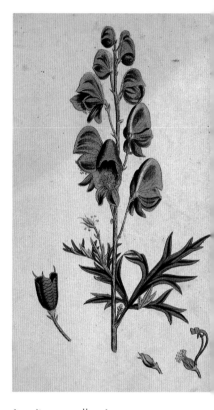

Aconitum napellus. *Lamson chose aconite because he had been taught that it was impossible to detect but, unfortunately for him, toxicology had advanced since he studied medicine.*

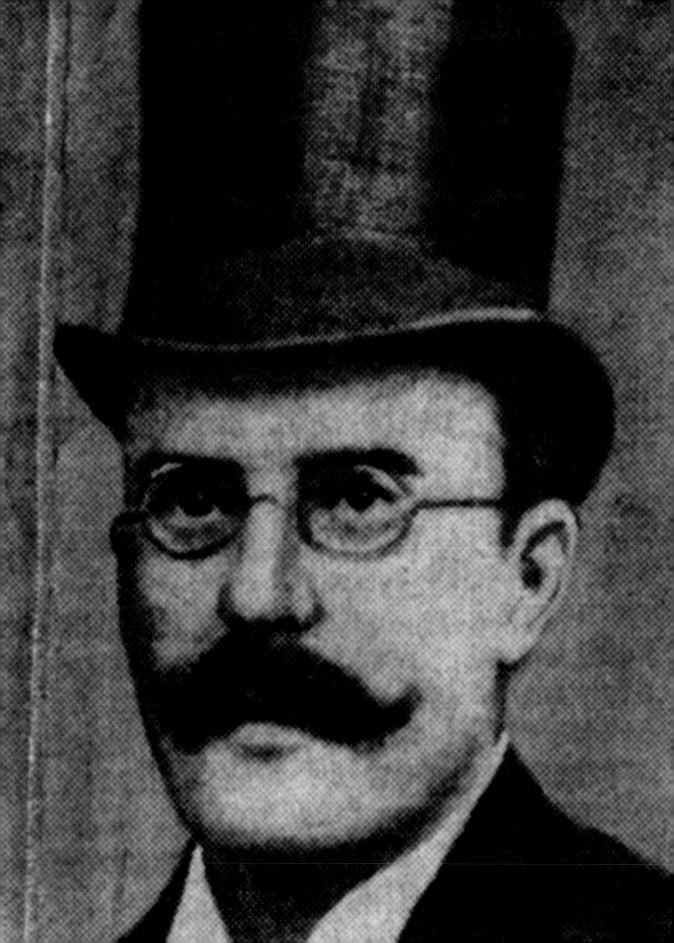

THOMAS CREAM
The Lambeth Poisoner

A graveside is an unusual place to find an accusation of murder. But one headstone in the tranquil Garden Prairie Cemetery, Boone County, Illinois, bears an oddly blunt epitaph: "Daniel Stott. Died June 12, 1881. Aged 61 years," and then—the punchline— "Poisoned by his wife and Dr. Cream."

D R THOMAS NEILL CREAM was at least as unusual as this inscription on the gravestone of his first proven victim. Nothing in his outwardly comfortable and respectable background seems to have marked him out as a future monster. Yet he was tried and convicted not once, but twice, and on both sides of the Atlantic.

A PROMISING YOUNG DOCTOR

Cream was born in Glasgow, the eldest of eight children. His parents emigrated to Canada when he was a small child, and the family settled in Quebec. Cream proved a good student at school, and his father, who worked as a lumber merchant, was financially comfortable enough for the teenage Thomas to attend McGill University in Montreal, where he studied pharmacology and medicine.

The young Thomas Cream was smart, tall, and handsome, although his good looks were marred slightly by a cast in one eye, just pronounced enough to be noticeable. He graduated from McGill with honors in 1876, having submitted a thesis on the subject of chloroform.

At this point comes the first suggestion that the agreeable young man may not have been quite what he appeared. He had been conducting a relationship with Flora Elizabeth Brooks, the daughter of a respectable hotel owner, and when she became pregnant, Cream performed an abortion on her. She was very ill afterward, and the doctor called to attend her told her father the true cause. No sooner had she recovered than the couple was marched up the aisle by the bride's infuriated father.

Cream did not stay by his new wife's side for long. Shortly after the enforced marriage, he set off back to Britain with the declared intention of gaining further

> "He wore gold-rimmed glasses and had very peculiar eyes ... as far as I can remember, he had a dress suit on ... he spoke with a foreign twang..."
>
> Lou Harvey, at the inquest into the death of Matilda Clover

Dr Thomas Neill Cream. *At the time of his arrest, Thomas Cream was still to all appearances a respectable member of society. But as the London police began to delve into his past, a very different image began to emerge.*

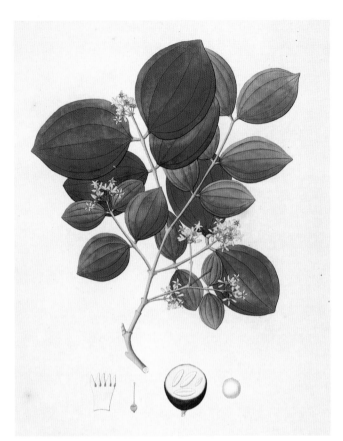

medical qualifications. He left Flora some medicine to remember him by, but it does not seem to have done her much good; she died, allegedly of tuberculosis, in August 1877. Subsequent events would mean that it was inevitably suspected that she had been Cream's first victim, but the body was never exhumed and nothing was ever proved.

Over in London, Cream briefly attended medical school, but left after less than a year and headed north to Edinburgh, where he joined the Royal College of Physicians and Surgeons. By 1878, he held a license in midwifery.

The Strychnos nux-vomica tree. *Flowers, foliage, and fruit of the* Strychnos nux-vomica *tree. The poison is extracted from the seeds and has a bitter taste, so it is often disguised in food or drink.*

THE FIRST DEATHS

After qualifying in Edinburgh, Thomas Cream headed back to Canada where he opened a practice in London, Ontario. He was soon known to offer abortions, then illegal, "helping out" women in trouble. In May 1879, Kate Gardener, who was known to have been his patient, was found dead in an alleyway behind his practice. She appeared to have overdosed on chloroform and an inquest was held. Her friend, Sarah Young, when questioned, said that Kate had gone to Cream to request an abortion, and that he had not only performed it, but had also suggested that Kate might blackmail her rich neighbor by accusing him of being her seducer. Cream did not emerge with much credit, but ultimately no case was brought against him, and very soon afterward he was on the move again—this time over the border to Chicago. Once there, he lost no time in setting up a new practice, conveniently close to the Levee District, the city's red light area.

Cream quickly became known for performing abortions, mostly on working girls, and sometimes with the help of a midwife, Hattie Mack. In August 1880, the body of Mary Ann Faulkner, a prostitute, was found in Mack's rented rooms. Mack was arrested and immediately accused Cream, who she said had first given Faulkner an abortion, then demanded Mack look after her when her recovery proved slow. Cream was charged with murder and put on trial, but defended himself by counter-accusing Mack of having performed the botched abortion. The accusations from both sides were lurid, but in the end Cream got off. He would not be so lucky when it came to the treatment of Daniel Stott.

AN AFFAIR AND ITS CONSEQUENCES

Cream spent a good deal of time experimenting with drugs, and in 1880 began to place advertisements in the Chicago papers claiming that he could offer a successful treatment for epilepsy. Daniel Stott, an epileptic, lived with his much younger wife, Julia, in Belvidere, about 70 miles (112km) from Chicago. On seeing the advertisement, Julia traveled into the city to consult Cream and collect the advertised drug for her husband. And at first it seemed to work—Daniel had fewer fits, and Julia returned for repeat prescriptions several times. Soon she had begun an affair with the attractive doctor. And in June 1881, Daniel died.

The death was at first attributed to a fit. But Cream sent telegrams to the coroner mentioning poison, and was eventually traced and questioned. As he had also suggested that Julia file a lawsuit against the pharmacist who had fulfilled the prescriptions, it seems likely that his ultimate aim in raising the question of poison was blackmail. However, while he may have been relatively efficient as a poisoner, Cream was a terrible blackmailer. In this case, the plan backfired badly.

Daniel Stott was exhumed, and his body was found to be full of strychnine. Cream, having stupidly drawn attention to himself, was accused of murder. At his trial, Julia sang like a canary in the witness box. He had seduced her, she said; she had seen him opening and refilling the pills she later gave to her husband—not only that, but it was Cream who had suggested blackmailing the unfortunate chemist. The jury believed her, and Cream was sentenced to life for murder.

JAIL, AND A RETURN TO LONDON

Thomas Cream's father had disowned him when he was first charged with the murder of Daniel Stott. But after his son had served ten years in prison, William Cream died. Thomas's brother, who had continued to support him

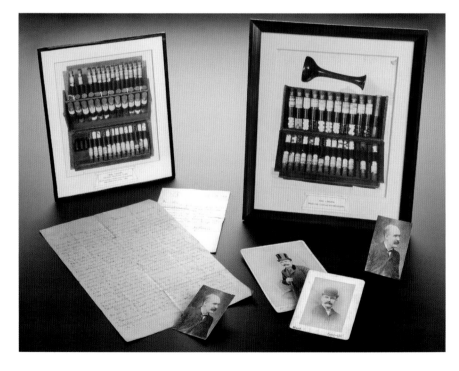

Memorabilia from the Cream case. *Part of Scotland Yard's collection of items from the case, including one of Cream's inept blackmail letters, and photographs showing his large collection of poison vials and of "people of interest," including one of Cream himself.*

while he was in jail, now worked hard to get the life sentence commuted, and ultimately—possibly with the help of bribes paid from the estate of their father—he succeeded. In the summer of 1891, after a decade behind bars, Cream was released from the Illinois State Penitentiary. By October, he was back in London, in lodgings at 103 Lambeth Palace Road, going by the name of Dr Thomas Neill.

> "He became a sensualist, a sadist, drug sodden and remorseless, a degenerate of filthy desires and practices."
>
> The Canadian Medical Association Journal,
> *reporting on the trial of* Dr Cream

The Thomas Neill who emerged from prison was older and distinctly more odd than the Thomas Cream who had been convicted in 1881. His squint was more noticeable and he was addicted to a mixture of powerful drugs including morphine and cocaine. He buttonholed strangers—men and women—in public houses, engaging them in rambling conversation and sharing his stash of pornographic photographs after even the shortest acquaintance. Gone was the urbane and authoritative doctor; someone much more sinister was emerging.

Three years earlier, the London slum area of Whitechapel had been the location of the notorious Jack the Ripper murders—all the victims were prostitutes—which had never been solved. As a result, when more murders started to take place in similarly impoverished Lambeth, also of prostitutes but this time using poison, the unknown killer acquired his own nickname: the Lambeth Poisoner.

First to die, on October 13, was 19-year-old Ellen Donworth. She had had an assignation with a "topper" (street slang for a man in a top hat—which indicated a gentleman), who had offered her a drink from a bottle he carried. She was found fitting in the street, gave her scant account of what happened to a policeman, and died as she was being taken to hospital. She had been given strychnine. Cream sent an anonymous letter to the coroner offering to identify the murderer in return for 300,000 pounds (several million dollars today).

On October 20, it was Matilda Clover's turn. She, too, was found in agony after having a drink with a tall, mustached gentleman. Clover, however, was in an advanced state of alcoholism, so her death was at first attributed to natural causes and as a result no autopsy was performed.

Various anonymous letters to rather random addressees began to arrive (Cream was up to his old tricks—but had become no more skilled at blackmail than before). Most of the recipients took them straight to the police. In November, "Dr Neill" disappeared, while Dr Cream paid a visit of some months' duration to his relatives in Canada. But he was back the following April, with

"I AM JACK…"
For years, a rumor persisted that Cream had confessed, moments before being hanged, to being Jack the Ripper. The hangman, James Billington, claimed that, as the noose was being placed over his head, he had called out "I am Jack…"—before the trapdoor beneath his feet opened and he was terminally interrupted. Appealing though the idea might be, Cream was still in prison back in Illinois when the Ripper murders were taking place in London—contemporary reporters believed that the most likely explanation was that Billington was adding some creative license to enhance his final account of Cream's death.

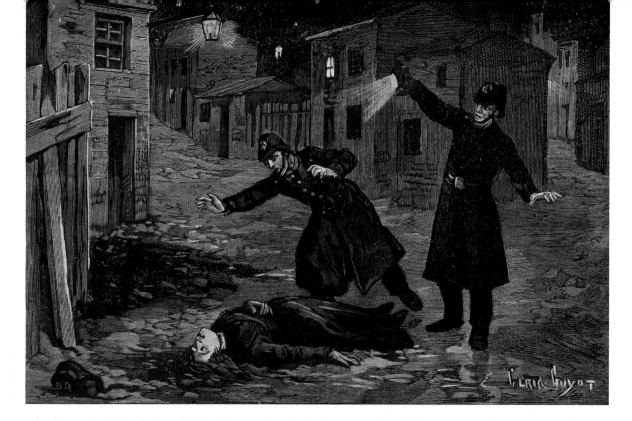

a fresh supply of strychnine obtained from a chemist in Saratoga, New York. On April 2, he made his only failed attempt at poisoning when he met a girl named Lou Harvey and gave her pills to take. She pretended to oblige, but threw them into the Thames instead and lived to tell the tale—and would prove to be Cream's nemesis on the witness stand. On April 11, Alice Marsh and Emma Shrivell, young prostitutes who lived in the same lodgings, were found screaming in the hallway by their landlady. Both died, but not before they had told her that they had gone out together with a tall gentleman with a moustache—with whom they had shared a drink.

Cream's next encounter was not with a prostitute but with a detective—a man named John Haynes, whom he met at a photographic studio where both men were waiting to have their portraits taken. They fell into conversation about the Lambeth Poisoner and the helpful doctor took his companion on a tour of the locations where the victims had lived and died. He seemed to know a lot about the case, but baffled Haynes by taking him to visit the lodgings of Matilda Clover—at that stage, not one of the known poison victims. Haynes shared his information with Sergeant Patrick McIntyre, an acquaintance with links to Scotland Yard, who found that Cream was already under surveillance as a "person of interest" as the result of his many convoluted attempts at blackmail.

Things finally started to pick up pace. Matilda Clover's body was exhumed on May 5, and by May 23 there was evidence that she had died from strychnine poisoning. In early June, Cream was charged with blackmail and extortion. In handcuffs, he attended the inquest into Clover's death, where he was amazed to see Lou Harvey, whom he believed he had murdered, risen from the dead to give powerful evidence against him, which would be used at his trial. Finally, in July, he was charged with Clover's murder. His trial took place three months later, and on October 21, 1892, the jury took only ten minutes to convict him. Sentenced to death, he was hanged, unrepentant, at Newgate Prison just three weeks later.

Finding a victim of Jack the Ripper. *At one point, Cream was also suspected of having been the Whitechapel murderer. But he had been behind bars when the earlier murders took place, and even the keenest conspiracy theorist could not place him at the scene.*

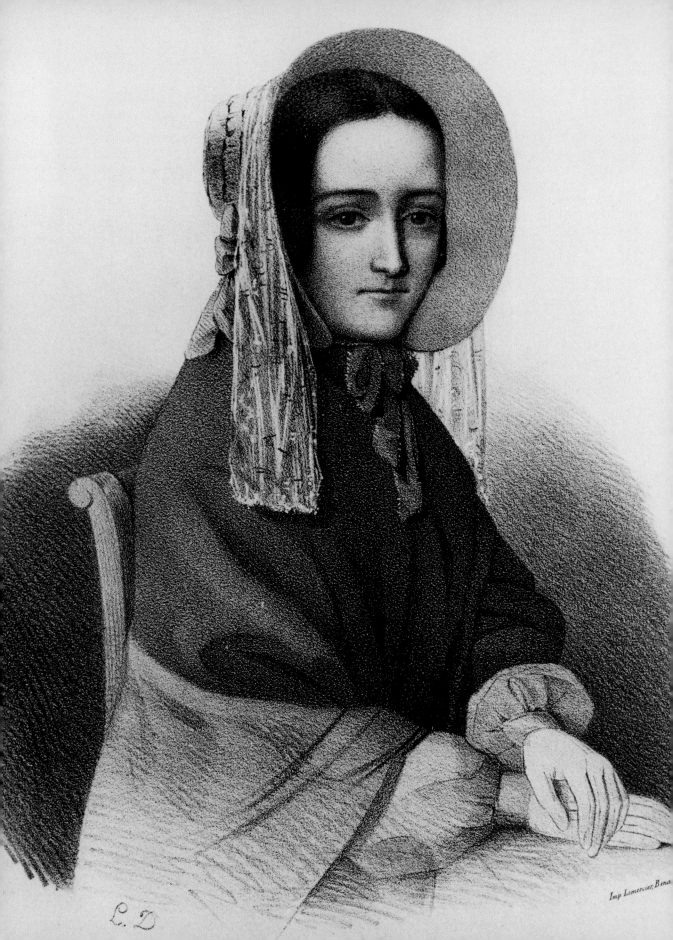

Imp Lemercier, Bena

MARIE LAFARGE
and the Marsh Test

Mary Blandy's trial (see page 66) may have been the first in which early forensics played a part, but it was the trial of Marie Lafarge that finally put forensics at center stage. Before the Lafarge case, the focus of guilt always turned on motive and access—did the person suspected have a reason to commit the crime, and, in practical terms, could they have done it? But a case in which scientists claimed they could prove a poisoning was still big news in the early 1840s.

ADD A WELL-BORN, attractive suspect with a taste for the dramatic, plus the backstory of an unhappy marriage in a Gothically bleak country mansion—not to mention a range of twists and turns that dragged the trial out for a very long time indeed—and it is hardly surprising that the Lafarge case was the OJ Simpson-style sensation of its day.

LIFE BEFORE MARRIAGE

Marie Cappelle was born to be disappointed. She came of a good family—her mother was the daughter of Monsieur Collard, who had held the esteemed post of Quartermaster General of the Republic, while her father was a career officer who had been a member of the Imperial Guard of the Emperor Napoleon and who later commanded a large garrison at Valence. She was educated, too—with the daughters of other distinguished families, she had attended the convent of St Denis, where she had become friendly with a number of girls of high rank and large fortunes. By the time she was in her late teens, she had a refined bearing, well-schooled manners, and the usual collection of drawing-room accomplishments of a young lady of her day. She also had a modest fortune of her own. At this point, though, her luck ran out. Her father was dead; he had been killed in a hunting accident when she was only 12, and her mother remarried but died herself a few years later when Marie was 18. The newly orphaned Marie was sent to live with her worldly aunt, Madame Garat, her mother's sister, who found the girl a trying companion, dreamy and impractical, and felt that she had been overindulged. She was keen to see her niece married, but although over the next five years she paraded Marie in front of all the eligible young men of the day, none

Marie Lafarge. *Popular engravings show a pale, refined-looking young woman, hair severely dressed under a heavily veiled bonnet, white-gloved hands serenely resting one on another. Could this ladylike creature really be guilty of murder?*

of them took the bait. It seemed that Marie was never quite rich enough, pretty enough, or appealing enough to be chosen over the rich, pretty, appealing girls by whom she was surrounded; somehow, she never seemed to be some fortunate young man's first choice.

Monsieur and Madame Garat decided that a match must be made by stealth. Privately, and without telling the girl, they consulted a matrimonial agent and challenged him with finding her a husband. Before long, he put forward a possible candidate: Charles Pouch Lafarge.

MARRIAGE AND THE JOURNEY TO LIMOUSIN

At the time he met Marie, Charles Lafarge was 28 years old. He was a heavy, awkward young man, not endowed with particularly appealing manners. However, he had been presented to the Garats as the proprietor of an iron foundry—a profitable career at a time when railways were starting to be built all over Europe—and the matchmaker told Marie's aunt and uncle that he also lived in a handsome château, Le Glandier, in the Limousin region in central France. The young couple were introduced at a concert, and while Marie's immediate impression was that her prospective husband was both plain and provincial, her relations ensured that she heard only of the advantages of the match—the fact that Monsieur Lafarge had fallen in love with her the moment their eyes met, the pretty house and rich estate that awaited her in Limousin, and the gorgeous trousseau with which she could equip herself before the marriage took place.

Spurred along by her relatives' enthusiasm, Marie agreed to the proposal. On August 10, 1839, the couple was married, and three days later they arrived home at Le Glandier. The homecoming was a terrible shock to Marie. Far from the commodious, well-appointed château she had expected, the house was dilapidated, with no modern conveniences or elegances, and sited next door to the smoky, dirty iron foundry. It was dreary, damp, and overrun with rats. It was obvious that the young bride had been duped; far from being rich, the family was

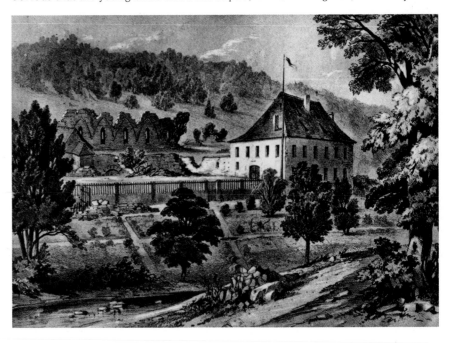

Not as advertised. *Bleak and run-down, Le Glandier must have been a highly unwelcome wake-up call for Marie. But she eventually seemed to make the most of her new situation—for a month or two, at least.*

POISON CABINET

Like so many others of her day, Marie's chosen poison was arsenic. During the first half of the nineteenth century it had become a popular instrument of murder—so much so that its nickname was "inheritance powder." Largely thanks to the Marsh test, it fell out of favor over the next few decades; as soon as it was possible to prove the presence of arsenic, it lost much of its value to those who wished to see off an inconvenient friend or relative quietly, without detection.

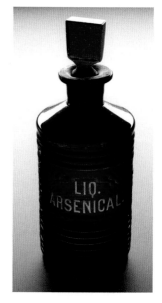

Arsenic. *Rats were a problem for many households in the nineteenth century—housekeepers didn't think twice about using arsenic to get rid of them.*

evidently barely getting by. She was greeted by her mother-in-law, whom she at first mistook for the housekeeper—Charles Lafarge's mother spoke in an accent so strong that Marie could hardly understand her, and seemed little inclined to indulge the pampered young Parisian.

That night, Marie locked herself in her bedroom and wrote a letter to her new husband, protesting at her betrayal and claiming to be in love with someone else. It begged him to release her from the marriage. Charles received it with dismay, but persuaded her to stay at least for a little time—things would improve, he promised, they just needed putting in order.

Reluctantly Marie began to take her place as chatelaine at Le Glandier. Charles's mother gave way to her, rather resentfully, and allowed Marie to arrange things more to her own liking. Refined meals were ordered, and Marie had them served in a daintier fashion than favored by her in-laws. Her husband bought her a piano, which she played in the run-down salon at the château. And she also made a friend, a niece of Charles, Emma Pontier, whose gentle manners (and admiration of Marie's Parisian élan) seemed to invite confidence.

CHARLES LAFARGE FALLS ILL

After about three months of marriage, Charles had to go to Paris on business. He wanted to register a patent in relation to his iron smelting business which he was convinced would finally render it profitable. By now, Marie seemed to have accepted the status quo in the marriage; she wrote him affectionate letters, and sent him a package of the local cake of which he was fond. Charles opened the parcel and ate a little, but that night he was seized by terrible cramps and vomiting; assuming that it had gone bad on its journey, he threw the rest of the cake away. The sickness lingered; he was still feeling fragile when he returned home in December and, after a delicate meal of chicken and truffles that Marie prepared to welcome him back, he was very ill indeed.

When summoned, the doctor thought that Charles had simply overeaten and brought on indigestion, but in the ensuing days the patient became steadily worse, although he was dosed with everything that either his wife or his mother could think of. At night, the couple could hear the rats running about in the eaves and along the rafters of the decrepit old house. Marie asked the servants to get her some arsenic, to be mixed with flour and water, and the resulting paste was laid about the corridors and in corners

"The small quantity of arsenic requested ... had not been enough to exterminate our little colony of rats; they had become still more odious to my husband." —From The Memoirs of Madame Lafarge, *published in English in 1841*

with the idea of getting rid of the vermin. The rats remained as lively as ever, but Charles's health had gone into a steep decline. Marie fed him chicken broth and gum arabic, which she said was a proven cure for digestive maladies. His family had become suspicious and tried to banish her from the sick chamber, as well as telling Charles to take nothing to eat or drink from his wife; Emma, Marie's only remaining friend in the household, warned her that they were gossiping about poison. And after suffering for a month with headaches, cramps, and nausea, Charles Lafarge died on January 16, 1840.

ARREST AND TRIAL

Ten days after Charles's death, Marie was arrested and, tearfully protesting her innocence, was taken into detention at nearby Brives. At the time of his death, no fewer than four doctors were attending Charles. They tested samples of the

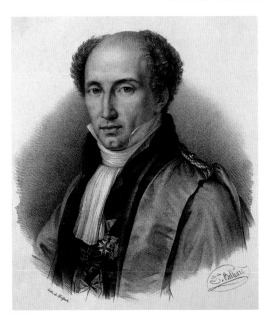

chicken broth he had drunk and found that it was thick with arsenic; they also tested samples of the rat-killing paste around the house and found that it consisted only of flour and water. Whoever had been taking the arsenic, it had not been the rats.

What followed was an extraordinary display of professional one-upmanship between Marie's lawyers and those acting for the prosecution. Charles's stomach had been removed before interment and local doctors carried out tests for arsenic—and found it. On hearing this evidence, Marie fainted in court—she certainly knew how to put on a good show, and by now the case was being followed in the press all over France. The prosecution called for tests to be carried out on other organs from the body, using the Marsh test, to be sure, and so, on orders of the judge, what was left of Charles Lafarge was exhumed in front of a large and interested crowd. Parts of the rotting internal organs were then tested for arsenic in a public outdoor laboratory watched by dozens of onlookers, many waving smelling salts underneath their noses—but no arsenic was found.

Mathieu Orfila. Aged 53 at the time of Marie's trial, Orfila was an academic, chemist, toxicologist, and author of A Treatise on Poisons, *which is still regarded as a classic in the complicated field of forensic medicine.*

THE MARSH TEST

Marie could be said to have been unlucky—the Marsh test, judged the first reliable forensic test for arsenic, had only just been developed at the time of her trial. It was named for its creator, a young British chemist called James Marsh. After failing to prove the presence of arsenic in a famous case in which the poisoner later admitted guilt, he had become determined to invent a failsafe proof. The favored test in the early nineteenth century involved making a solution of the material believed to contain arsenic and passing hydrogen sulfide through it. If it contained arsenic, the mixture would then turn yellow; the problem was that the yellow coloring faded within an hour or two, so the proof could not be used for a jury. In 1840, Marsh devised a test to replace it, in which the sample was heated with acid and zinc; the resulting gas, if arsenic was present, left a deposit that had a powdery, silver appearance—and it was stable, allowing it to be kept and shown in evidence. The Marsh test continued to be used until the 1970s.

The relief Marie must have felt did not last long. The prosecutor, worried that the locals were not meticulous enough in applying the new test, now insisted that the acknowledged world expert in toxicology, a man named Mathieu Orfila, must come from Paris to offer his opinion. After lecturing the court on the perfect way to carry out the Marsh test, Orfila conducted it once again on the, by now surely rather sparse, remains of Lafarge. In keeping with the dramatic reveal, a huge thunderstorm broke overhead as he delivered his verdict. And this time arsenic was found. After months of suspense, on August 30, 1841, Marie Lafarge was found guilty and given a life sentence of hard labor. She had to be carried from the courtroom.

AFTERMATH

From beginning to end, the gathering of evidence against Marie and the trial that followed had taken almost a year. Public opinion for and against her had ebbed and flowed, and, like all defendants in all notorious trials, she gained a fan base, much of it consisting of young men who wrote and proposed they "save" her by marriage. While she waited to be tried, she wrote a dramatic popular memoir, stressing her innocence, which became a bestseller not only in France but, upon swift translation, in England and America, too. Still, there was no happy ending for Marie. She would serve 11 years in prison, but her health, never very robust, broke down under the harsh regime, and, suffering from tuberculosis, she was eventually freed in June 1852. She took modest lodgings in Ussat, a quiet town in the far southwest of France, but died in November, barely six months after her release.

"Madame Lafarge was brought into court on Thursday, in an arm-chair, so pale and weak that she seemed scarcely alive." —*Extract from the journal of Thomas Raikes,*

contemporary commentator on the trial

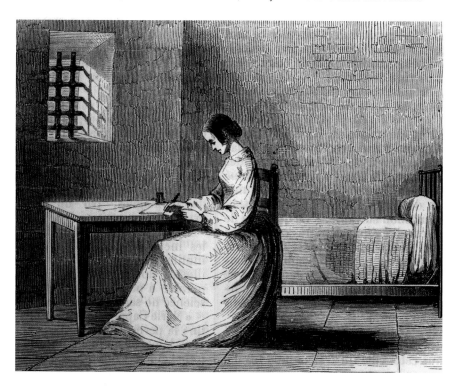

In prison. *Locked up for nearly a year awaiting trial, Marie wasn't idle; The Memoirs of Madame Lafarge, a self-penned lengthy declaration of her innocence, was in print within six months.*

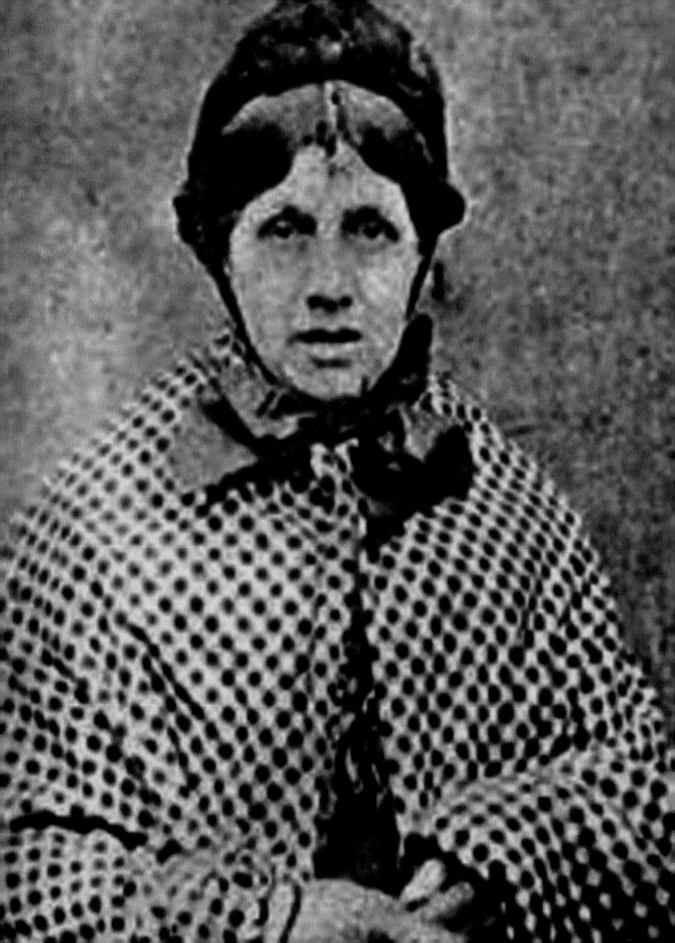

MARY ANN COTTON
The Dark Angel

In Victorian Britain, the era that heralded modern "health and safety" awareness, there were two lingering factors that almost cried out to a would-be murderer to try the dark art of poisoning: the prevalence of arsenic in everyday objects and the inadequacy of the sanitation system. And one woman, dubbed the Black Widow, would take full advantage of both.

MARY ANN ROBSON was born—or so it is believed, in the absence of a birth certificate—on October 31, 1832. Her birthplace was Low Moorsley, a small village in the English county of Durham, but the family later moved to the coal-mining village of Murton. Her father died in the mine when Mary Ann was ten years old, and ten years later she herself married a miner—and made her first acquaintance with the joys of life insurance.

MARY ANN'S MARITAL HISTORY

Mary Ann and her first husband, William Mowbray, had eight or nine children, all but one of whom predeceased their father. In January 1865, Mowbray too died, leaving Mary with a life insurance payout of £35 (around $45), around £3,000 ($4,055) today—a large sum for a working-class woman, equivalent to about six months' wages for a manual laborer at the time, which Mary Ann used to embark on a career in nursing. She dispatched her one remaining child to live with her parents and took up a position in a hospital where she met husband No 2, George Ward, an engineer. They married in August 1865, only months after William Mowbray's death, and just over a year later Ward, too, died. Once again, Mary Ann benefited from the life insurance.

Husband No 3 was at first Mary Ann's employer, a recently widowed shipwright named James Robinson, with whom she took up a position as housemaid the month after Ward's death. Soon afterward, one of Robinson's children died. While she was still an employee, Mary Ann visited her mother, who was ill and died within days, and when Mary Ann returned to work, bringing her one remaining daughter with her, the daughter and two more of Robinson's children died. But despite the fact that Mary Ann was starting to look like the kiss of death personified, she became Mrs Robinson and gave birth to two more children, one of whom died in babyhood.

Mary Ann Cotton. *Her blank expression belies the fact that in her younger years she was described as strikingly beautiful.*

Robinson himself, however, remained alive and well—and observant. He noticed, for example, that money was missing from his bank account; that valuable items were disappearing from the house (he learned that his wife was coercing his older children into pawning them); and that Mary Ann was overly keen for him to take out life insurance for himself and his children. Marriage No 3 ended in Mary Ann's undignified dismissal from the marital home. It is thought that she took to living on the streets—but not for long.

> "I saw him have fits, he was very twisted up and seemed in great agony. ... He said, 'It is no fever I have.' ... I have seen (Mary Ann) several times give him a drink."
>
> *Eyewitness to the death of Joseph Nattrass*

BIGAMY AND BEYOND

There was no divorce from James Robinson, but this did not prevent marriage No 4 from taking place—bigamously—in September 1870. The "groom" was Frederick Cotton, the widowed brother of Mary Ann's friend Margaret, who had been caring for Frederick and his two children but had died in March of that year. Frederick died in December 1871, leaving Mary Ann with his two existing children, a third on the way, the proceeds of his life insurance, and his surname, which she retained to the end of her life. By July 1872, all three children would be dead.

Mary Ann lived next with Joseph Nattrass, a man with whom she is thought to have had affairs during her second marriage and the fourth, bigamous marriage. He died in April 1872, shortly after revising his will in favor of Mary Ann. The last man in her life, and father of the last of her many children, was an excise officer, John Quick-Manning. This very last child was born in Durham—or to be more precise, in Durham Jail.

THE COMMON FACTOR

It might appear that Mary Ann's family life was doomed to be characterized by natural death, punctuated as it was by the frequent demise of husbands and children—until one takes a closer look at the nature of those deaths and discovers a common theme. William Mowbray and all but one of his children died of gastric fever, as did George Ward. One of James Robinson's children died of gastric fever and two more, along with Mary Ann's mother and Mowbray's surviving child, apparently died of hepatitis, the symptoms of which are very similar to gastric fever. Margaret Cotton died of an unidentified stomach ailment—gastric fever?—and her brother Frederick died of gastric fever, as did his three children. Joseph Nattrass, too, died displaying symptoms of gastric fever.

This somewhat vaguely named disease was indeed rife in Victorian Britain—but could one woman really be so unlucky as to lose husbands, children, and stepchildren to that one illness, when there were so many other diseases

THE FINAL TALLY
Even had she been found not guilty of Charles Edward Cotton's murder, there were plenty of further charges lined up for Mary Ann to answer—she is believed to have murdered up to 21 people in total. These were: three husbands, a lover, her mother, her best friend, a number of stepchildren, and most of her own children.

to claim the lives of Victoria's subjects? Was it possible that Mary Ann, apparently immune to gastric fever, was systematically bumping off her nearest and dearest using arsenic? The symptoms of arsenic poisoning are, after all, almost identical to those of gastric fever.

ARSENIC IN VICTORIAN BRITAIN

Victorian Britain enjoyed the fruits of the Industrial Revolution, at its height in the nineteenth and early twentieth centuries—and so too did arsenic. As a by-product of the purification process of metal ores such as iron, copper, and tin, all of which were in great demand, white arsenic trioxide was sold by enterprising industrialists as rat poison. But on a more subtle level, arsenic, combined with sulfur or copper, was used to produce dyes in the rich reds and greens beloved by Victorians, and thus was literally everywhere: in clothing, candles, toys, and most significantly in the heavy wallpapers that graced the walls of Victorian homes. The flour and water paste used to hang the wallpaper promoted the growth of mold, which in turn processed the arsenic into a gas and released it for Victorian families to inhale at leisure.

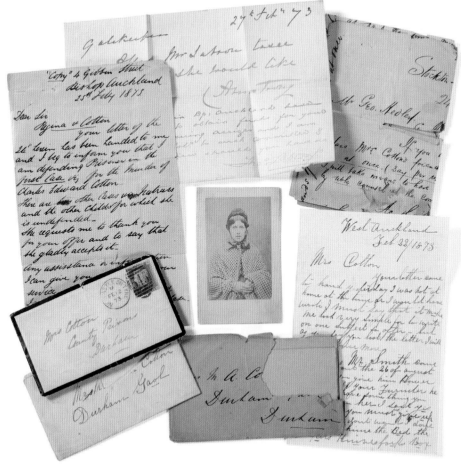

Correspondence. *These letters, from and about Mary Ann, surfaced only recently, an anonymous donation to Beamish Museum, County Durham. They were written while she was awaiting her execution.*

GASTRIC FEVER

In Victorian Britain, gastric fever was largely the result of poor sanitation in the increasingly populated towns and cities, and poor hygiene on the part of their citizens. Had Mary Ann lived on to continue practicing her dark art, it would have been more difficult to pass off the symptoms of arsenic poisoning as gastric fever, as there was a major overhaul of the country's sanitation system in the second half of the nineteenth century. It began in London, inspired by the "Great Stink" of 1858, when the River Thames was so awash with raw sewage that members of parliament sitting in their debating chamber beside the water feared the noxious odor alone would kill them off.

Another factor was the expansion of the British Empire and the increase in ocean-going traffic—especially with the introduction of steamships—to countries in Asia, exposing merchant seamen to virulent diseases such as cholera. Mary Ann's first husband, William Mowbray, worked for a short time as a fireman aboard a steam vessel.

DEATH BY TEAPOT

Arsenic in its most toxic form, arsenic trioxide, is a rather "genteel" poison beloved of the famous crime writer Agatha Christie as a murder weapon. It is colorless and dissolves readily in liquid, making it easy to administer in drinks—and Mary Ann Cotton, British through and through, is thought to have poisoned her victims via tea poured from her small, black, trusty Wedgwood teapot (now on display at Beamish Museum, County Durham). Her last request before her execution was, predictably, for a cup of tea.

MARY ANN MAKES A MISTAKE

Astonishingly, no suspicion fell on Mary Ann until the death of Frederick Cotton's seven-year-old son, Charles Edward, in July 1972. Had all the deaths occurred in one small village, eyebrows might have been raised much sooner, but in the course of her several marriages Mary Ann had moved from the northeast of England to the southwest, then back to various locations in the northeast. In any case, regulation of the sale of arsenic had only recently been introduced, and record-keeping was lax. And, of course, it was perfectly normal in Victorian times

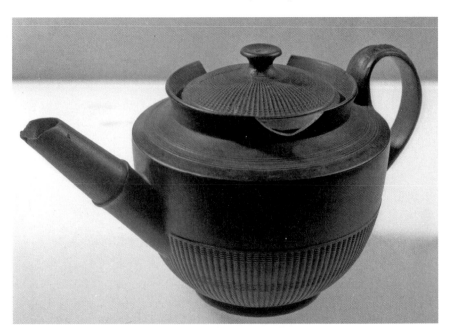

A quintessentially English murder weapon. *Mary Ann's Wedgwood teapot, made by the famous pottery Josiah Wedgwood and Sons.*

for children to die in infancy or childhood—they were lucky to live past the age of five—and life expectancy was a mere 45 years for a middle-class man, and only half that for the working classes. Poor sanitation, poor hygiene, and poor nutrition added up to a poor prognosis.

But a throwaway remark was to place Mary Ann's head in the hangman's noose. During a conversation between Mary Ann and one Thomas Riley, a parish official in the village where she was living, Riley asked whether she and John Quick-Manning were planning to marry. And Mary Ann (skimming over the fact that Quick-Manning was already married) replied that she couldn't marry him because of her remaining stepson, Charles Edward, adding cheerfully, "T'won't matter, I won't be troubled long." She quickly justified this odd statement by pointing out that the Cottons were not a long-lived family. Shortly afterward, Charles Edward was dead.

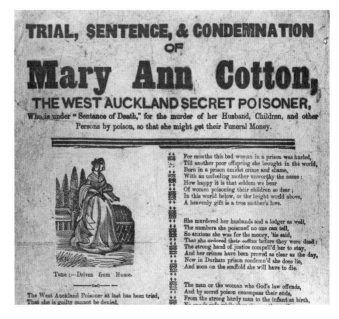

Trial report. *"The West Auckland Secret Poisoner"—a sensational report of Mary Ann's trial.*

GUILTY AS CHARGED

The local doctor carried out a hasty postmortem and declared the probable cause of death to be gastric fever. But when Thomas Riley recounted his conversation with Mary Ann, the contents of the child's stomach were examined more closely using the Reinsch test—a pioneering method devised in 1841 for detecting the presence of heavy metals—and enough arsenic was discovered to have killed five men, let alone one small boy. The game was up for Mary Ann! She was arrested and imprisoned in Durham Jail, awaiting the birth of the baby she was expecting, to be followed by her trial. John Quick-Manning, the baby's father, disappeared, leaving Mary Ann to face her fate alone.

The baby, Margaret, was born in early January, 1873, and Mary Ann was allowed to nurse her for ten weeks before handing her over for adoption (Margaret died in 1954, at the impressive age of 81). The trial lasted three days. Mary Ann protested her innocence, and her court-appointed defense lawyer did his best to persuade the jury that the culprit was not Mary Ann but the arsenic emanating from wallpaper. The jury were unmoved by his eloquence and after only an hour of deliberation unanimously found her guilty.

THE END OF MARY ANN

Mary Ann's execution, carried out on March 24, 1873, was witnessed by some 20 reporters, who had plenty to say on the matter. "Mrs Cotton," wrote a journalist from the *Dundee Courier*, "who scowled fiercely and with an air of defiance at the crowd, and who muttered constantly but indistinctly, took her place upon the drop with remarkable composure." But there was to be one last drama before Mary Ann was "launched into eternity"—there was not enough of a drop below the trap door to snap Mary Ann's neck in the noose, so the hangman, William Calcraft, had the grisly task of pressing down on her shoulders until she succumbed to death.

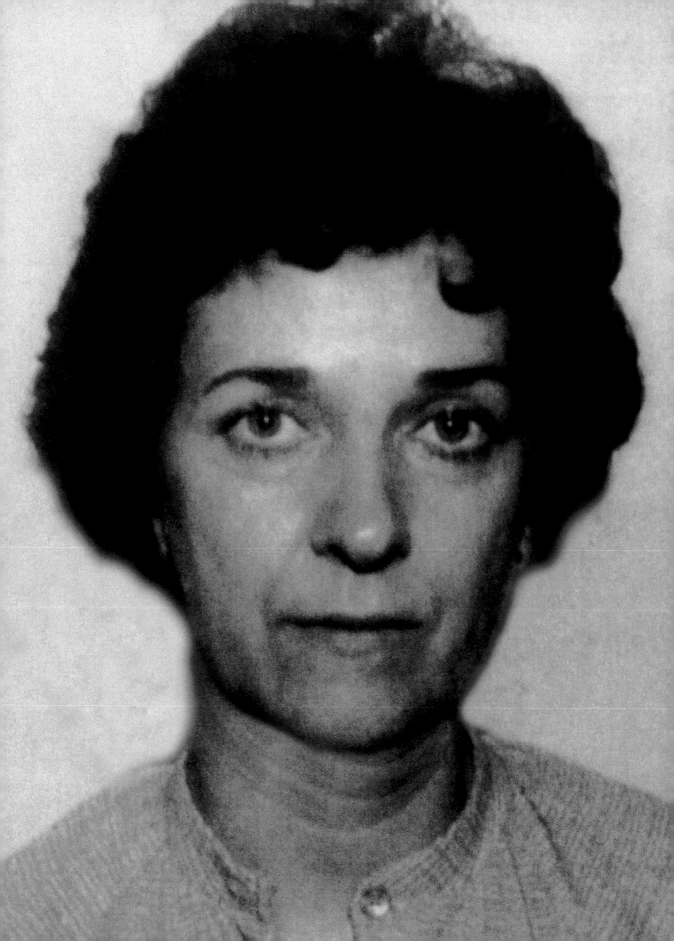

AUDREY MARIE HILLEY
The Runaway Poisoner

The plump, disheveled woman resting outside a house on the outskirts of the small mill town of Blue Mountain in rural Alabama on a wintry afternoon in February 1987 looked tired and ill. Concerned homeowners found her sheltering on their outside deck, but her responses to their questions were incoherent. Eventually they established that her name was Sellers and that she had been looking for help after her car broke down, but she was soaking wet and freezing cold—in fact, she looked as though she'd been outside for days, not hours.

AN AMBULANCE was called, but "Mrs Sellers" began fitting on the way to the hospital and died from the effects of hypothermia later that afternoon. And those who found her had been right to be suspicious. The dead woman's real name was Audrey Marie Hilley, she was a convicted murderer, and the police had been hunting for her for several days.

The death made headlines in the local press. One of the people who found Hilley, Janice Hinds, had grown up with her, but still had been unable to recognize her. "That woman was pitiful," Janice told the local press. "We didn't know she was Marie Hilley. She didn't look like Marie Hilley. Marie was a sophisticated lady. She had pride in her looks, her dress."

A BELLE OF ANNISTON

Janice's memories of Marie as a real southern belle had their roots in childhood. Marie's parents, Huey Frazier and his wife Lucille, did not have much money and worked long hours, but they had aspirations for their cute, smart daughter. Within their limited means they spoiled Marie, indulging her when she threw tantrums and encouraging her to dress and behave like a lady. They wanted a white-collar future for her; when, in 1951, she married a high-school friend, Frank Hilley, at the age of 17, it was probably something of a disappointment. Frank was in the navy, and he was steady enough—and besotted with Marie—but he had a similar background to her own and he certainly was not rich. Still, while he was serving abroad, he faithfully sent home his earnings, and when

Mistress of disguise. *Attractive and audacious, Audrey Marie Hilley was a risk-taker. She took on several identities to suit her purposes, including that of her own—nonexistent—twin sister.*

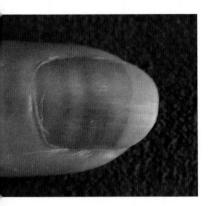

Telltale sign of poisoning. *When the Aldrich-Mees' lines appear in the fingernails, it is a reliable symptom of an overdose of arsenic.*

he left the navy a couple of years later, he quickly found work as a shipping clerk. Meanwhile, Marie worked as a secretary, and gave birth to a son, Michael, in 1952, and a daughter, Carol, in 1960. They looked like a perfect family, but cracks began to form in the marriage after the first year or two.

Marie was a spendthrift; she loved nice clothes, and fancy furniture and decorations for the home, but not budgeting. She also insisted that the family move to a house on McClellan Boulevard, a major thoroughfare and one of the nicer streets in Anniston, even though it was really beyond their means. From quite early on in their relationship, Frank suspected her of being unfaithful. Marie's parents moved in with the couple in 1962, and Lucille helped her daughter with childcare. Three years later Marie's father, Huey, died, but Lucille stayed on with the Hilleys. Tensions in the house remained, but the marriage managed to limp on through the 1960s and into the early 70s. Michael left home and went to college, while Carol turned into a tomboy teenager, apparently constantly at odds with her mother over her choice of sporty clothes and her dislike of wearing frills or makeup—her refusal, in fact, to be more like Marie herself.

THE END OF THE MARRIAGE

On May 19, 1975, Frank Hilley visited his doctor to report terrible stomach cramps, rapid weight loss, and constant nausea. The doctor prescribed medicine for a stomach infection. When Frank got home, Marie began to administer injections—shots that she said contained Phenergan, a medicine against nausea recommended by the doctor. At around the time of the first doctor's appointment, Frank called his son Michael in Florida and said he needed to talk to him in person, but the meeting never took place and Michael never discovered what his father had wanted to tell him. Frank became increasingly unwell. On May 23 he was taken to hospital, where he died two days later. The diagnosis—and ultimate cause of death—was given as acute hepatitis.

Frank had had a life insurance policy of just over $31,000—a substantial sum in the mid-1970s and Marie was the named beneficiary. The money allowed her to buy a new car, new clothes, and presents for the rest of the family, and to make plans to redecorate the house. But when the insurance money ran out, Marie began to write dud checks.

A CHAPTER OF DISASTERS

Over the following three years, things became difficult for Marie and she accused a number of her neighbors of harassment, ranging from housebreaking to threatening phone calls. The local police department received repeated calls from her, which they took seriously and with which they tried to deal, but after following up numerous lines of inquiry they always seemed to result in dead ends. By 1979, Marie was writing increasing numbers of bad checks and was trying desperately to cover up her lack of money. She had also taken out a life insurance policy on her daughter, Carol, in 1978, with Marie as the named beneficiary.

In August 1979, Carol was admitted to hospital as an emergency. She was being violently sick and was in terrible pain. But the doctors were unable to find the cause. She was sent home briefly, but was soon back in hospital, accompanied by her frantic mother, who begged the doctors to find out what was making her so ill. By early September, Carol had lost dramatic amounts of weight and was complaining of numbness in her hands and feet. The medical staff had begun to question if the symptoms were psychosomatic. Later it would transpire that Marie, apparently so desperately upset by her daughter's condition, was giving her secret shots of "medicine" that she promised Carol would bring about a cure.

Luckily, before her mother's injections could kill her, a sharp-eyed doctor noticed whiteish ridges on Carol's fingernails. Known as Aldrich-Mees' lines, these are classic symptoms of arsenic poisoning, so she was tested for arsenic levels. As Marie waited at the hospital for news, the police arrived and she was arrested—not for poisoning first her husband and then her daughter, but for bouncing nearly $7,000 in checks all round town.

With Marie under arrest, and very high levels of arsenic found in Carol, people began to remember Frank's death four years before. In retrospect, his symptoms had been quite similar to Carol's—and an exhumation and postmortem showed that he had easily enough arsenic in his body to have killed him. Marie was already in detention, and her story proved to have plenty of holes when she was questioned in detail. On October 25, she was charged with the murder of Frank, the attempted murder of Carol—and with passing dud checks. Ironically, one of them had been the payment for Carol's life insurance policy; even if her daughter had succumbed to Marie's ministrations, Marie would have found that she was unable to collect.

> "She'll be living a good life. She will be in a beauty shop at least twice a week."
>
> *Anonymous* FBI *agent quoted in the local press at the time of Marie Hilley's first disappearance*

Marie's odyssey. Marie Hilley *eluded capture for many years in an odyssey that stretched from Texas to Vermont.*

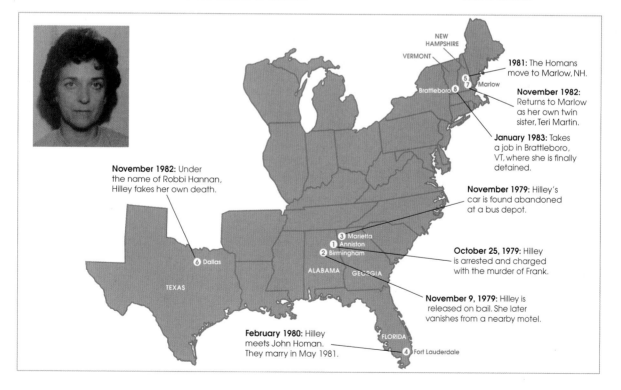

1981: The Homans move to Marlow, NH.

November 1982: Returns to Marlow as her own twin sister, Teri Martin.

January 1983: Takes a job in Brattleboro, VT, where she is finally detained.

November 1979: Hilley's car is found abandoned at a bus depot.

October 25, 1979: Hilley is arrested and charged with the murder of Frank.

November 9, 1979: Hilley is released on bail. She later vanishes from a nearby motel.

November 1982: Under the name of Robbi Hannan, Hilley fakes her own death.

February 1980: Hilley meets John Homan. They marry in May 1981.

NEW HAMPSHIRE
VERMONT
Brattleboro
Marlow
Marietta
Anniston
Birmingham
Dallas
ALABAMA
GEORGIA
TEXAS
FLORIDA
Fort Lauderdale

MYSTERIOUS MOTIVE

Marie's passing left many questions unanswered. There seems to be little doubt that she murdered for money. But that does not explain the different personas she took on, nor the elaborate Robbi/Teri charade.

Perhaps what Marie craved most of all was to escape from her humble beginnings and have some drama in her life. Yet she was buried in a grave alongside that of Frank Hilley, the husband she had poisoned; despite all her efforts, she was unable to escape the confines of Anniston in the end.

FLIGHT, AND TWO NEW IDENTITIES

Marie was given bail, but she had no intention of sticking around for a trial; in mid-November, she simply disappeared. Her car was found in Georgia but there was no sign of Marie herself, and the police in Alabama were to hear no more of her for some time.

In February 1980, a man named John Homan met an attractive woman at a bar in Fort Lauderdale, Florida. She told him that her name was Robbi Hannan, and they began dating. He was recently divorced and quite shy, but she seemed to find him appealing, and by May 1981 they were married. Shortly afterward, they moved to New Hampshire, where they both found jobs, Robbi as a secretary at the Keene Screw Company.

In her new role as Robbi, Marie became a fully fledged fantasist. She regaled coworkers with a dramatic life story that included dead children, an identical twin sister called Teri, and a mysterious illness. The latter became the main theme of the tales she told throughout 1982; it was degenerative, it would be fatal, she was going to pursue some last-ditch hopes for treatment in Texas, where her sister lived. Her colleagues were sympathetic, and her new husband seemed to believe every word she said. When she took off for Texas in the fall of 1982, he waited for news. At first, he had the occasional call from Robbi, but in early November he heard from her sister, Teri, with some shocking news. Despite Robbi's brave fight against her illness, Teri told him, it had finally got the better of her and she had died. Devastated by Robbi's loss, Teri wanted to come to New Hampshire to see her late sister's husband and the friends she had made there. And the following day Teri Martin, 50 pounds thinner than Robbi, a snappy dresser with bleached-blonde hair, met John at the airport and went home with him.

Could John really have thought that Teri and Robbi were two different women? It appears that Marie did convince him. When police later tracked Marie's movements over the three months she had been away, they found that she had stayed in Texas for only a day or two before returning to Florida, where she worked, in the Teri Martin identity, as a secretary in Pompano Beach. She had told her coworkers and boss at her new company all about her sick twin sister.

Neighbors and colleagues of the late Robbi were not as credulous as John Homan. There were some difficult conversations and one ex-colleague of Robbi's told "Teri" frankly that she didn't believe her. "Who are you?" she is said to have asked, but Teri bluffed it out and stuck to her story. She stayed with John (so they could "grieve together") and took a job at a printing company in Brattleboro, Vermont, just over the state line. Meanwhile, some of the coworkers who had not swallowed her story began looking into Robbi's alleged death in Texas. They quickly found that the various stories that Teri had told failed to add up, and someone called the police.

CAUGHT AT LAST

Early in January 1983, Teri Martin was visited by police officers. They asked her who she was, and—for once—she told the truth. She was Marie Hilley, she admitted—she was wanted by the court back in Alabama. What for? Passing bad checks, she said. Back home she lodged an innocent plea on the charges of murder and attempted murder and her lawyers did their best to discredit the witnesses, particularly Carol, but it didn't work—the jury took less than half a day to convict her. She was given a life sentence for murdering Frank Hilley, and 20 years for the poisoning of Carol Hilley. On June 9, she as admitted to the Julia Tutwiler Prison for Women to begin her sentence.

Marie was a well-behaved prisoner. She maintained contact with Carol and with John Homan, who still seemed to believe in her, despite having known her with no fewer than three different identities. Two years after she began her jail term, she was trusted enough to be allowed out for the day. In February 1987, she was granted her first 48-hour break, and she left prison to spend it with John in Anniston, her home town. But on February 24, Homan called local police to tell them that Marie had vanished from the motel where they were spending her furlough. She had left a note telling him that she had gone, and that he should not expect to see her again. But it was only a couple of days later that she was found in a dreadful state on Janice Hinds' back porch. Lieutenant Gary Carroll, one of the officers who had interviewed Marie after Carol's illness and Frank's death and who had learned the hard way about Marie's escapology skills, thought that something must have gone wrong with her plan. "Normally, she's got an elaborate plan and can pull off a smooth escape," he said. "This time, it was spur of the moment and she got desperate." Marie was taken to hospital suffering from exposure and hypothermia. She was pronounced dead just over three hours later.

> "She wanted a high-rolling lifestyle; Frank's wasn't enough."
>
> *Joe Hubbard, assistant district attorney*

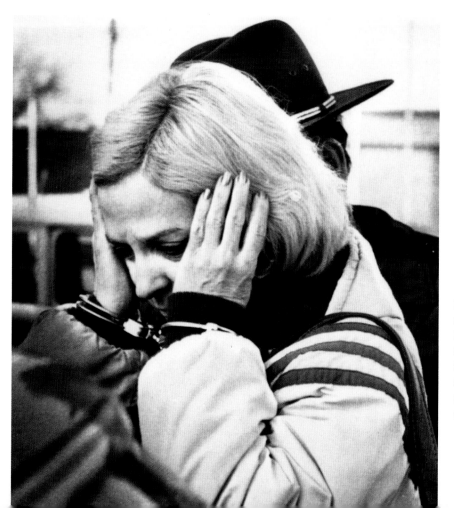

Blonde bombshell. *Marie snapped on her way to court. Her naturally dark hair had been dyed fair for her Teri Martin impersonation. Stress hadn't led her to neglect her manicure; as usual, despite the circumstances, she was impeccably presented.*

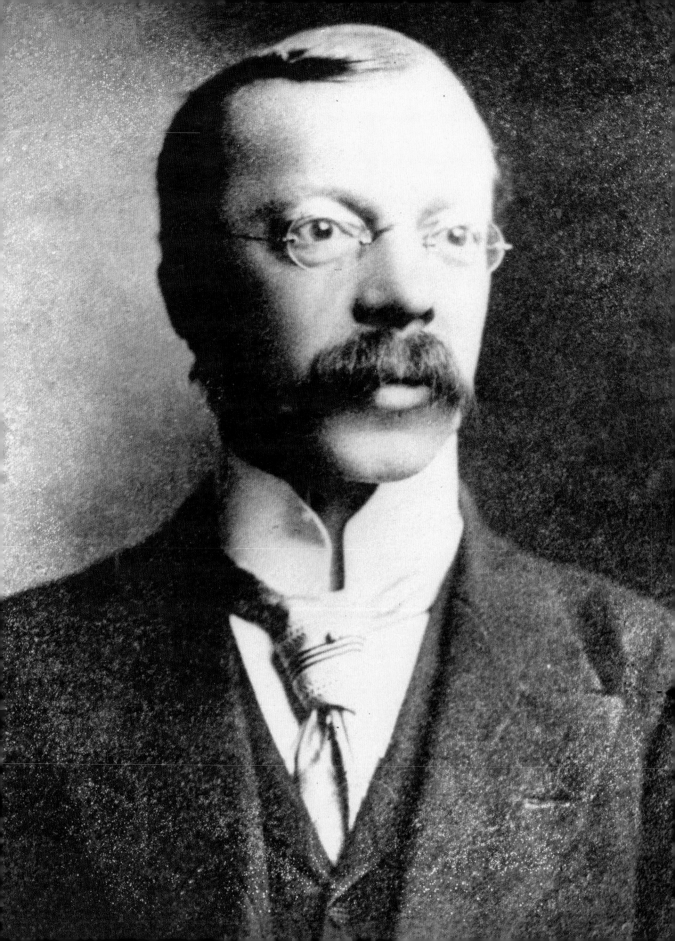

DR CRIPPEN
The Gentlemanly Poisoner

"Mild-mannered," "unassuming," and "kind": rarely can a poisoner have been described in such positive terms. And it's one of the oddities of the case of Hawley Harvey Crippen that he attracted so much sympathy, even from the hardened gentlemen of the press. After all, despite his modest appearance, the gentle-looking little man in the dock had killed his wife. It was not until nearly a century after his execution that some intellectually curious scientists questioned whether he actually had.

POISONER

Hawley Harvey Crippen
Born: September 11, 1862, Coldwater, Michigan, USA
Died: November 23, 1910, Pentonville Prison, London, England
Motive: To escape his marriage and make a new life with his mistress
Poison: Hyoscine
Number of victims: 1

MYRON AND ANDRESSE CRIPPEN were storekeepers in Coldwater, Michigan. Well-off and devoutly Protestant, they brought up their son Harvey in comfortable surroundings, and ensured he was both a hard worker at school and a regular worshiper in church.

Harvey initially lived up to his parents' expectations, taking a place at the University of Michigan. However, he left university in 1883 without completing his medical degree. He appears to have had a taste for travel and spent a brief period in England, working at a major psychiatric hospital. Returning to the United States, he joined the Cleveland Homeopathic Medical College, from where he graduated in 1884. He relocated to New York to specialize in ophthalmology at the New York Ophthalmic Hospital. He left with another degree in 1887.

Dr Crippen stayed on in New York for a while, working as an intern at the Hahnemann Hospital, where he met and married a nurse, Charlotte Bell. They moved to San Diego, but tragedy struck when Charlotte fell ill and died in January 1892, midway through her second pregnancy—the couple already had a baby son, Otto. Harvey Crippen found juggling a career with the demands of bringing up a young child impossible, and delivered Otto to his grandparents to look after before returning to New York.

The early 1890s were not as easy economically as the 1880s had been, and Crippen found that life in New York had become tougher. Nevertheless, he found a job with Munyon's Homeopathic Home Remedies, working on formulating the company's products. He did well there, and was promoted twice—first to their Philadelphia office, and then again when he was given the job of opening offices in England, in Liverpool and London.

Dr Hawley Harvey Crippen. Well-brought-up in middle-class circumstances, many of Crippen's friends and supporters refused to believe he could be guilty of murder.

THE DOCTOR AND THE SHOWGIRL

Crippen did not remain a widower long. In New York his path crossed that of Cora Turner, an aspirational actress and singer aged just 19, more than a decade his junior. The pair married in September 1892, just eight months after the death of his first wife.

Was it the glamor of the stage that attracted him? And could it have been the idea of financial steadiness and a comfortable home life that appealed to her? While Harvey Crippen was slight, quiet, and reserved, Cora, whose parents were Polish—and whose birth name had been the considerably less American-sounding Kunigunde Mackamotski—was flamboyant, with a fashionably opulent figure and a lively manner. She had left home to make her own way aged 16, and used the stage name of Belle Elmore. When the two met in New York, Crippen was earning a high salary at Munyon's, more than enough to keep Cora in the style to which she wished to become accustomed, and to pay for singing and acting lessons.

The marriage started well enough, and Cora and Harvey moved to Philadelphia on his first Munyon's promotion and then in 1897 to London on his second promotion. For the next few years Cora did her best—not very successfully—to launch herself on the London stage. Contemporaries noted that, although she was enthusiastic, she was not very talented.

Meanwhile, Harvey's fortunes gradually dwindled. He lost his job toward the end of 1899—apparently at least in part because he had spent too much of his time trying to promote Cora's theater career—and took a position as a consulting doctor at the Drouet Institute for the Deaf. It was here that he became friendly with a quiet young girl who was working as a secretary. Her name was Ethel Le Neve, and she was only 17.

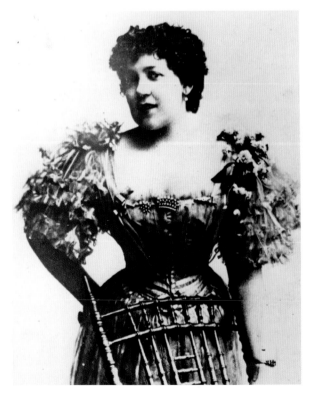

Cora Crippen, aka Belle Elmore. A *noisy, outgoing character, Cora seemed an unlikely mate for the reserved, quiet doctor.*

THE MARRIAGE FAILS

Ethel was very different from Cora and seemed a much more natural match for Harvey Crippen. The friendship progressed at a slow burn; meanwhile, the marriage between Harvey and Cora was going badly wrong. Some of this had to do with Harvey's reduced earnings. On their arrival in London the Crippens had lived in Piccadilly, but when he had lost his job they moved for a time to furnished rooms in the much dowdier district of Bloomsbury. Eventually,

> **BELLE ELMORE: A *VERY* MODEST TALENT**
> Cora, or Belle, had difficulty forging a career in vaudeville. Offers of stage time, even in the provinces, were few and far between. One story tells of her crossing a picket line to perform during a strike of artistes, upon which the noted English music hall star Marie Lloyd—who was supporting the strikers—acidly remarked that the pickets shouldn't worry, because Cora's performance would be bound to empty the theater anyway.

in 1905, they settled in Holloway, in north London, at 39 Hilldrop Crescent. It was an address that would be notorious before long.

Cora, always looking for an audience, had joined the Music Hall Ladies' Guild. She may not have been a successful performer, but her keen fundraising, tales of the New York stage, and habit of hosting small suppers at Hilldrop Crescent made her popular with the Ladies' Guild, and she was given the role as honorary treasurer of the guild. For a time, she and Harvey also took lodgers, and she is believed to have had affairs with one or more of them; one story had Harvey walking in on her in flagrante. On Cora's part, she suspected Harvey of having an affair, but didn't know with whom.

In 1908, Harvey Crippen entered a partnership with a London dentist, administering anesthetic, and Ethel joined him there, acting as the practice's secretary. The pair were now deeply in love, and Cora seems to have become fully aware of the situation toward the end of 1909.

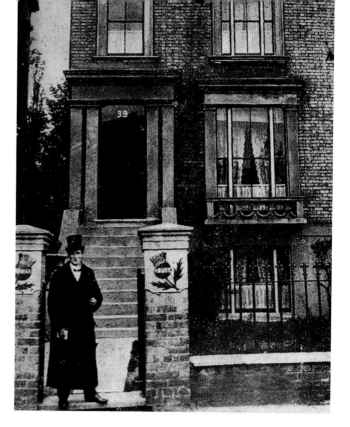

Scene of the crime. *In the 1920s and 30s, 39 Hilldrop Crescent would feature regularly in "House of Horror" press articles, but the house and its neighbors were flattened in 1942 in the course of a German World War II air raid.*

CONSEQUENCES

By late 1909, the Crippens were rowing constantly and events moved quickly. On January 19, 1910, Crippen collected some hyoscine hydrobromide from a pharmacy in Oxford Street. He had placed the order two days earlier for five grains, a huge quantity of a drug that was generally used in very small doses to calm the nerves or as a cure for nausea. On January 31, the Crippens entertained the Marinettis, stage connections of Cora's, to supper at Hilldrop Crescent. They had a pleasant evening, playing cards and chatting, and the guests did not leave until the small hours. It would be the last time anyone saw Cora alive.

On February 3, the secretary of the Ladies' Guild received a letter, purporting to be from Cora, resigning from her position as treasurer. It said that she had been called back to America to tend to a close relative, who was seriously ill. Later that month, Harvey attended a dance held by the Music Hall Ladies', but with Ethel Le Neve as his partner, a bold move which caused much disapproving tutting among Cora's friends. By early March, Ethel was openly living with Crippen at Hilldrop Crescent, and it was noticed that she was wearing items of clothing and jewelry that belonged to Cora.

The ladies of the guild were by now very worried about Cora and made constant inquiries of Harvey about when she would return. Perhaps it was this badgering that forced him into action; in any event, on March 24 he sent the Marinettis a telegram telling them that Cora had died, suddenly, in America. When he sent it, he was already en route to Dieppe, France, for a short holiday with Ethel. Increasingly unhappy with what they had been told, members of the Ladies' Guild had arranged for inquiries to be made in America about Cora. When they couldn't find anything out, her disappearance was reported to the police.

As a result, on July 8, Harvey Crippen had a visit from Chief Inspector Dew of Scotland Yard. He quickly admitted to the detective that he had been lying about Cora's absence; she had left him for another man, he said, and he had lied because

POISON CABINET

Hyoscine hydrobromide was an unusual drug of choice for a murderer. For one thing, unlike more everyday options, such as arsenic, it would have attracted more attention, necessitating a special order from the pharmacy—especially in large quantities. It is derived from plants of the deadly nightshade family; if Cora Crippen was killed by an overdose, she would have been aware of a dry mouth and possibly blurred vision before falling unconscious. If the overdose was large, she would have died shortly afterward.

In Crippen's time, small doses of hyoscine were used to reduce tremors (today, it is still a common treatment for Parkinson's Disease) and to calm a variety of stomach and bowel irritations.

he was embarrassed to be a cuckold. Chief Inspector Dew left, fairly satisfied by the explanation, but Harvey panicked. On July 9, he departed with Ethel for Antwerp, from where, on July 20, they caught a transatlantic liner, the SS *Montrose*, bound for Quebec, Canada. They passed themselves off as a father and son duo—Harvey became "Mr Robinson," while Ethel disguised herself in the outfit of a teenage boy.

> "Have strong suspicions that Crippen London cellar murderer and accomplice are among saloon passengers. ... Accomplice dressed as boy. Manner and build undoubtedly a girl."
>
> *Telegram sent by Harry Kendall, captain of the* SS Montrose

DISCOVERY—AND THE TRIAL

On July 11, Dew returned to Crippen's office. His intention seems only to have been to ask a few more questions to tidy up loose ends. But on discovering that neither Crippen nor Le Neve had turned up for work, he went to their home address and discovered the house in the process of being packed up, its owner already gone. Dew ordered a thorough search of number 39, and on July 13, the torso of a body was found buried in the cellar. The head, legs, and arms were missing—and were never recovered—and the torso had been "filleted," in other words, all the major bones had been removed.

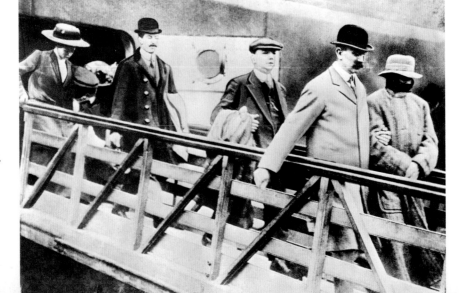

Arrested on board. Dr Crippen, his face concealed by a scarf, is led by Chief Inspector Dew down the gangplank of the Montrose.

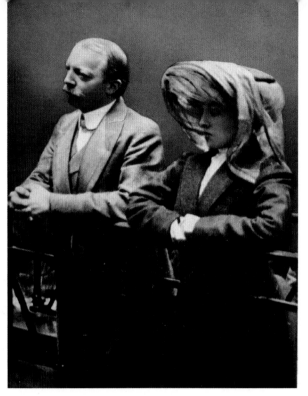

The call for Crippen and Le Neve's arrest went out immediately. Famously, the case was the first in which identification leading to arrest was made by the use of wireless telegraphy—Captain Kendall on the *Montrose* had already become suspicious of Mr Robinson and Ethel made an unconvincing boy. Chief Inspector Dew caught a faster boat, the SS *Laurentic*, which, despite leaving three days later, arrived in Quebec on July 30—the day before the *Montrose* was due to dock. The next day, as the *Montrose* neared port, Dew came on board and Crippen and Le Neve were arrested.

They were taken back to stand trial in London. By now, forensic examination had found 0.4 of a grain of hyoscine present in the remains, which it was estimated had been buried in the cellar for between six and eight months; the torso appeared to have been buried quite soon after death. A scar found on a piece of the flesh indicated an abdominal operation that matched Cora's medical history. The list of findings in the grave was both macabre and poignant. In addition to the main body section, a curler with hair in it, fragments of a human liver and kidney, and a pair of women's combinations were dug up, as well as parts of a pajama jacket that was identified as Crippen's own. In the four-day trial at London's Old Bailey courthouse, Crippen pleaded not guilty, and exhibited the gentlemanly behavior that won him some approval—he refused to implicate Ethel in any way. His refusal to confess and the condition of the remains meant that details of how the murder had been carried out could only be guesswork, although an overdose of hyoscine seemed the likeliest method. Unsurprisingly, given his purchase of the drug, the presence of hyoscine in the body, and the many lies he had told, the jury took less than half an hour to find Crippen guilty and he was sentenced to hang. As he had wished, Ethel was cleared—there was no real evidence that could show how much she had known about the murder.

Crippen was hanged at Pentonville Prison on November 23, 1910. Ethel visited him every day until his execution. The day after he was hanged, she left for New York, from where she traveled on to Canada, where she took up secretarial work once more before returning to England some years later. She eventually married and had a family; her children only found out about her involvement in the Crippen case when journalists came visiting after her death in 1967.

In the dock. *Crippen and Le Neve, the latter heavily veiled, stand side by side at the Old Bailey to hear the charges read against them.*

WAS CRIPPEN GUILTY?

In 2007, nearly a century after Crippen's execution, a team of American forensic scientists from the University of Michigan compared DNA from preserved fragments of the torso discovered at Hilldrop Crescent and found that not only did it not match that supplied by descendants of Cora, but also that it came from a male. Their findings have since been debated, but they raised an interesting question. Crippen was a very atypical poisoner, and had protested his innocence to the bitter end. Was there even the slightest possibility that he could have been telling the truth?

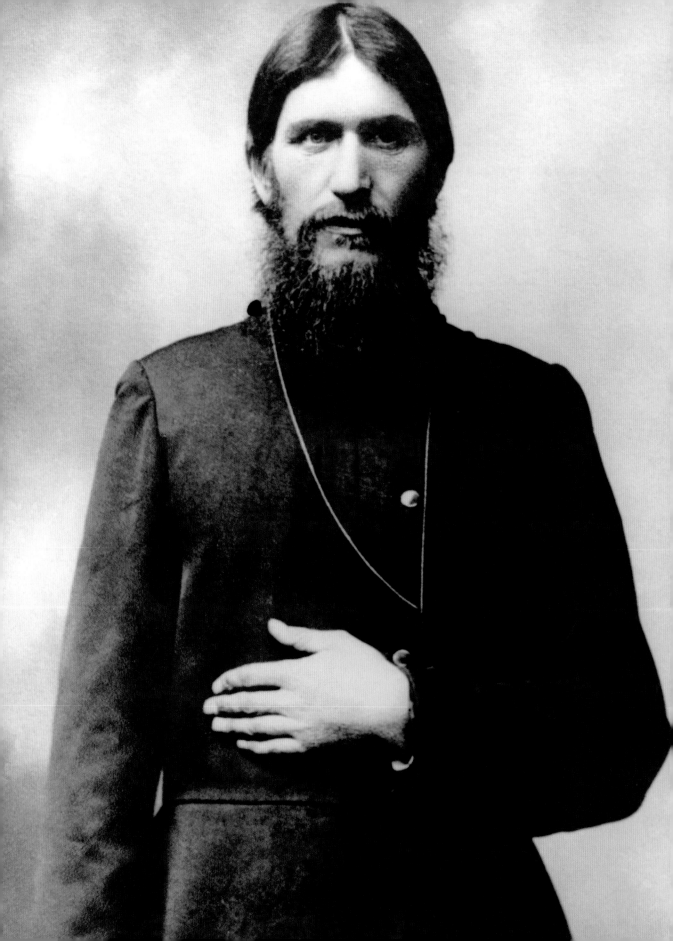

RASPUTIN
The Superhuman Monk

In the early twentieth century, an enigmatic character known as Rasputin became an unlikely favorite of Russia's czar and czarina. Within a few years, the world was at war, and while the czar was busy at the Eastern Front, Rasputin was exerting rather too much influence on the czarina—so Russian nobles hatched a murderous plan, making cunning use of the Mad Monk's fondness for beautiful women.

R ASPUTIN WAS BORN in around 1872 to a peasant family living in Pokrovskoye, a small village in the stark landscape of Siberia. His education was somewhat perfunctory and indeed he is thought to have been virtually illiterate all his life; but from early on he displayed signs of possessing mystical powers, and it was this facet that would shape his identity.

THE MAKING OF THE MAD MONK

When Rasputin was in his late teens, he spent several weeks in the monastery at Verkhoturye, a major center of Russian Christianity; but if he harbored ambitions to lead a cloistered monastic life they were never realized, although he would in time become known as "the Mad Monk." Instead, he married, had a son, and looked set to settle into contented fatherhood. However, the baby soon died and Rasputin threw himself into a religious frenzy. He pored obsessively over the Bible and in 1892 he set off on a pilgrimage on foot, first to Mount Athos in Greece, the spiritual center of Orthodox Christianity where Russian Orthodox monks have lived since the eleventh century, and from there to Jerusalem.

And at some point on this long and grueling trek, Rasputin morphed into the character with which the world has since become familiar—a bundle of nervous energy, oozing charisma, and with a strange intensity in his eyes, chilling yet compelling. Despite his somewhat unprepossessing image—filthy clothes on an unwashed body, a long, rough beard, and thin, lank hair—he gained a fine reputation as a starets, a wandering holy man and healer, who could predict the future. He also became

> "His gaze was at once penetrating and caressing ... direct and yet remote."
>
> *Maurice Paléologue, French ambassador to Russia*

Rasputin. *Pictured in 1910, the early days of his fateful relationship with the Russian royal family.*

known, rather more dubiously, as a "rasputnik"—a lecher. Although promiscuity appears at odds with Rasputin's profound spirituality, it was apparently his interpretation of the self-flagellation practiced by the Russian Orthodox Khlysty sect as a means of communing with the Holy Spirit. His seduction technique, to which many an aristocratic Russian woman would succumb, was to assure his quarry that sin was an essential step on the path to true repentance. Rasputin's wife, meanwhile, perfected the art of turning a blind eye to his infidelities, and remained devoted to him, producing several offspring, of which only three lived to adulthood.

This, then, was the wanderer who in 1903 arrived in St Petersburg—home of the Romanovs, the Russian royal family—and effectively changed the course of modern history.

MEET THE ROMANOVS

The Romanov dynasty was founded in 1613, the outcome of a period of instability known, ominously, as the "Time of Troubles." The dynasty was beset with succession problems, with the perpetual battle for the throne even ending, on one occasion, in assassination. By the time Czar Nicholas II acceded in 1894, the Russian people were becoming decidedly disenchanted with the social and political system imposed by their imperious emperors, and revolution was brewing.

Czar Nicholas was not constitutionally suited to the rule of a vast and problematic empire; he was, however, by nature a family man. He had married

The Romanovs. Czar Nicholas II with his wife and children. At the royal couple's feet is their son and heir, Alexis, the source of the Romanovs' close relationship with Rasputin.

Alexandra Feodorovna, a granddaughter of Britain's Queen Victoria, shortly after his accession. Like her ancestor, Alexandra was a formidable character but also a loving wife and mother, and Nicholas was devoted to her. Between 1895 and 1901, Alexandra gave birth to four daughters, and the couple were desperate for a son.

ENTER RASPUTIN

En route to St Petersburg in 1903, Rasputin visited the monastery at Sarov, once home to the renowned mystic Saint Seraphim. Here, Rasputin exercised his own mystical powers, predicting that a son and heir to the Romanov dynasty would be born within a year. And indeed Alexis, czarevitch of Russia, entered the world on August 12, 1904. However, Alexis had a potentially life-threatening congenital condition, carried through the maternal line from Queen Victoria: hemophilia. The lack of a coagulation factor in his blood meant that even the merest scratch became a traumatic event.

Nicholas and Alexandra doted on their son, and were beside themselves with anxiety. When Alexis was in the midst of a bleeding episode in 1908, his parents called in desperation upon Rasputin—who had been introduced to the family three years earlier—for help. And the child's health did indeed improve, seemingly miraculously, although with the hindsight of modern medical knowledge it seems quite likely that it was Rasputin's admittedly shrewd recommendation to stop administering aspirin, now known to have the effect of thinning the blood, that did the trick.

But miracle or not, the future of the royal family, and of Rasputin himself, was sealed, for the Mad Monk now held the czar and, even more significantly, the czarina completely in thrall. Focused only on the necessity to have Rasputin on hand to keep their son alive, they refused to believe reports of the Mad Monk's appalling womanizing, and those who dared to bring accusations against him found themselves banished from the royal circle. Nicholas faltered once, on reading a report of Rasputin's misdeeds provided by his prime minister, but Alexandra was so anguished at the prospect of Rasputin's expulsion that Nicholas capitulated and allowed him to stay.

Larger than life. *A caricature of Rasputin depicted on a magazine cover a few months after his death.*

RUSSIA AT WAR

On August 1, 1914, Germany declared war against Russia. Nicholas was by temperament far more comfortable with military conflict than the civil unrest that had been simmering persistently since 1905, when a minor revolution had led to constitutional reforms. In September 1915, he joined the Russian troops at the Eastern Front, taking personal command. Unfortunately, here too his shortcomings as a leader were in evidence, and faith in his ability to rule diminished even more.

Meanwhile, back in St Petersburg, Rasputin was not improving matters. Nicholas had left Alexandra in charge of internal affairs, with Rasputin as her personal advisor, and the nobility watched with increasing horror as his detrimental influence grew. Another, far more significant revolution was looming, and the Romanovs were unwittingly playing right into the hands of their disgruntled subjects. Only one thing could now save Imperial Russia: Rasputin must go.

WRONG CHOICE OF VEHICLE?

Only a small quantity of potassium cyanide, Dr Lazovert's chosen poison, is required to kill a person. However, Lazovert, more used to healing people than assassinating them, was perhaps unaware that when cyanide is administered in the presence of alcohol and sugar—in Rasputin's case, wine and petits fours—its efficacy as a murder weapon is reduced, since the cyanide reacts with the sugars to form amygdalin, which is a less toxic compound.

DEATH BY CYANIDE

The telltale smell of bitter almonds wafting from a victim makes cyanide poisoning fairly easy to identify. Another sign is the victim's blood turning from red to a deep Prussian blue, the result of iron in the blood binding to the cyanide ion.

Symptoms set in very quickly and progress from headache, nausea, and rapid heart rate to seizures, low blood pressure, slow heart rate, and cardiac arrest, with loss of coordination and hyperventilation thrown in for good measure.

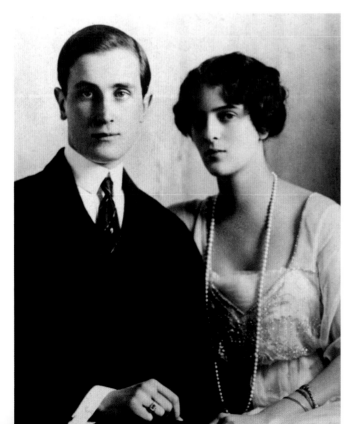

Prince Yusupov. One of the conspirators in the plot to dispose of the vexatious Rasputin, Yusupov is pictured here with his alluring wife, Irina.

AN INVITATION TO A WINE TASTING

According to the evidence of the conspirators in the plot to exterminate the human pest that was Rasputin, on the freezing cold night of December 30, 1916, he visited the Moika Palace at the invitation of Prince Felix Yusupov, the husband of the czar's beautiful niece, Irina. Yusupov had lived in London, where he had been the life and soul of fashionable society, so he knew how to throw a good party, and of course the prospect of meeting the lovely Irina was a huge enticement to Rasputin.

Present at the gathering, along with Yusupov, were Vladimir Purishkevich, a politician and staunch monarchist; Grand Duke Dmitri Pavlovich, the czar's cousin; Dr Stanislaus de Lazovert, a close friend of Pavlovich; and Sergei Sukhotin, an army officer. To Rasputin's disappointment, Irina was not there—he could not know that she was only ever intended to be a lure. Nor could he know that in preparation for Rasputin's visit, Dr Lazovert had donned a pair of surgical gloves and crushed to a fine powder crystals of potassium cyanide, a highly poisonous compound with a smell reminiscent of almonds, the main ingredient of petits fours....

What greeted Rasputin was a small table upon which sat a selection of rare wines, and two plates of petits fours. The cakes on one plate were flavored with chocolate, and those on the other with rose. Had he been on his guard, Rasputin would have noticed that the other guests only sampled the chocolate petits fours. This was a sensible move, since the filling in the pink cakes had been sprinkled with a dose of cyanide sufficient to kill "a monastery of monks" instantly. Rasputin tucked into the pink cakes with gusto, and enjoyed several glasses of wine from bottles also heavily laced with cyanide. He was having a wonderful time—but why wasn't he dead?

DESPERATE MEASURES

Rasputin's would-be assassins were at a loss. Yusupov later reported that they were "seized with an insane dread that this man was inviolable, that he was superhuman, that he couldn't be killed." The poison apparently hadn't done a thing except to make Rasputin belch, and the only option was to shoot him. But even this was not as straightforward as it should have been; the first shot, aimed straight at his heart, left him momentarily writhing in pain, but then he somehow staggered to his feet and made a bid for freedom. Two more shots were fired into his retreating back, and his assassins, satisfied that the Mad Monk was finally dead, hastily wrapped his corpse in a sheet and lobbed it through a hole in the icy waters of the Neva River. Divers retrieved the body on January 1, 1917.

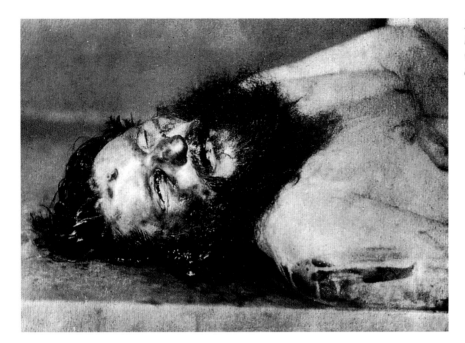

A reign of terror ended. *The battered body of Rasputin after he was pulled from the freezing waters of the Neva River.*

DEAD WITHIN TWO YEARS

Appropriately for someone with Rasputin's reputation for accurate prophesy, he foresaw the nature and outcome of his own death: "If I die at the hands of the Russian people, the Czar and his descendants will be safe for centuries. If I die at the hands of the aristocracy, this Neva River will run red with their blood, and the Czar's family will all be dead within two years."

And he was of course right; although the UK's *Manchester Guardian* reported after Rasputin's death that "Russia breathes more freely for the removal of a most baleful influence," its optimism was premature. The Russian Empire collapsed in early 1917, following the first of two revolutions that year. Czar Nicholas II abdicated on March 15 and a provisional government was established. The second revolution, known as the Bolshevik Revolution, established Russia's Soviet Communist government, and on July 17, 1918, the czar, his wife, and their five children were brutally slaughtered by Bolshevik forces.

The remains of Nicholas, Alexandra, and three of their daughters were recovered in 1991 and reburied in a state funeral in 1998; but it was not until 2007 that the bodies were recovered of the fourth daughter and of Alexis, their precious son whose longed-for birth had led to the family's ill-fated association with Rasputin, dubbed "the blackest devil in Russian history."

"Without Rasputin, there would have been no Lenin." —Alexander Kerensky, head of the *provisional government*

FACT OR FICTION?

The postmortem on Rasputin's body revealed that there were no traces of poison, and that the cause of death was a shot in his forehead—so it's possible that the assassins' account of his death was heavily embellished to demonstrate how dangerous he was, or that Dr Lazovert lost his nerve and instead of cyanide had secretly laced the petits fours with a harmless substance.

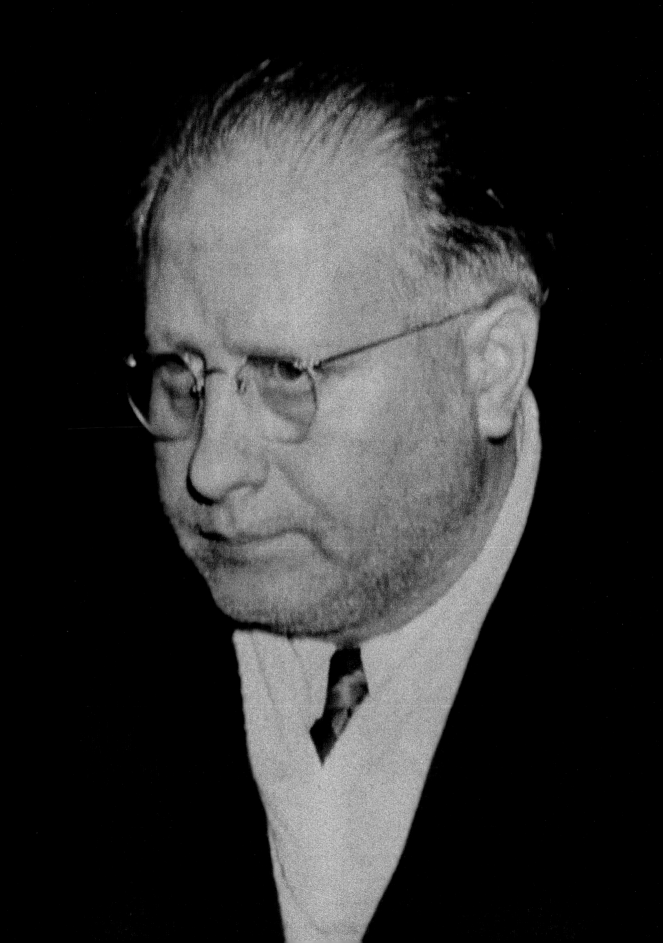

THE PHILADELPHIA POISON RING

The 1929 Wall Street Crash saw America transformed from the Land of Opportunity into the Land of the Great Depression, and while many found themselves homeless and eating out of soup kitchens, others devised new ways to generate income. Among these were two Italian cousins who, along with their cohorts, discovered there was profit to be made from manufacturing … widows.

POISONER

Herman and Paul Petrillo
Born: Date unknown, Italy
Executed: 1941, Philadelphia, USA
Motive: Financial gain
Poison: Arsenic
Number of victims: At least 70

THE LATE NINETEENTH and early twentieth centuries saw Italian immigrants flooding into the United States to escape the poverty and hardship rife in their homeland. Between 1900 and 1910 alone, around two million Italians set foot on American soil to start a new life, including our two cousins, Herman and Paul Petrillo. They headed to Philadelphia, where they both set up in business—Herman as a spaghetti salesman and Paul as a tailor. And when the Depression began, they added more lucrative sidelines— Herman in counterfeiting and Paul in insurance scams.

THE DEPRESSION SETS IN

The end of the 1920s saw a period of economic prosperity in the United States coming to an end. Unemployment was rising, real estate values were falling, and Europe had slapped a tax on the import of surplus industrial and agricultural goods from America in a tit-for-tat response to an American act, passed in 1922, that imposed duties on foreign imports. The stock market, however, was enjoying an unprecedented boom, mainly the result of short-term investment by speculators buying on margin through brokers such as small banks. But in 1929, the market began to fluctuate wildly, going from an all-time high in early September to a flurry of panic selling in late October. Reinvestment by a group of bankers restored confidence, but it was a temporary fix and on October 29, 1929—a date forever to be known as "Black Tuesday"—over 16 million shares were sold, adding to the almost 13 million disposed of just a few days earlier. Combined with the already weakened economy, it was disastrous. Many failed to recover their investment; banks and businesses closed, and the unmitigated misery of the Great Depression was underway.

> "Gentlemen, you are about to witness the death of an innocent man."
>
> *Herman Petrillo, shortly before his execution*

Paul Petrillo. *Tailor, con artist, counterfeiter, joint proprietor of a matrimonial agency—and ruthless murderer.*

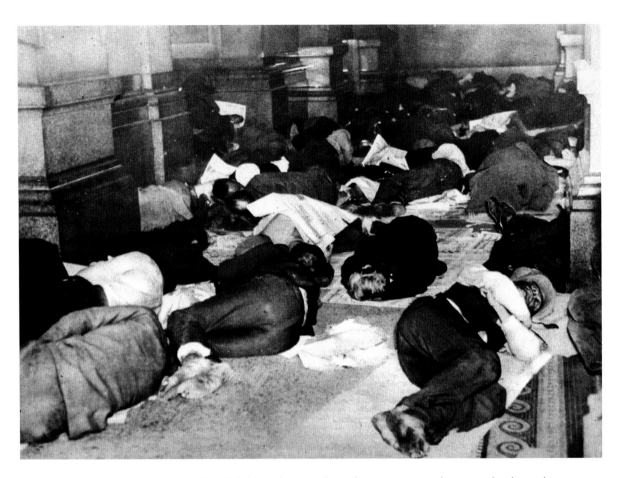

The Great Depression. *In stark contrast to the creature comforts born of the economic boom of the 1920s, the early 30s saw many Americans taking shelter wherever they could find it.*

Philadelphia—the city where the country's Declaration of Independence and Constitution had been signed, and the Liberty Bell hangs as a symbol of freedom—was in a particularly poor state owing to the dogged determination of its leaders to reject federal aid in favor of going it alone. The citizens responded with strikes, marches, riots, and demonstrations, but to no avail, they continued to suffer while the rest of the country benefited from the relief program. This was not the life Herman and Paul Petrillo had signed up for; they had not come to the United States only to be plunged back into the hardship they'd left behind—so they decided to start a matrimonial agency. Because love is what makes the world go around, right? Wrong. *Money* makes the world go around.

THE MATRIMONIAL AGENCY

On the face of it, the enterprise set up by the Petrillo cousins and a third man, Morris Bolber, was no different to any modern dating agency targeting a specific audience. Their raison d'être was to find lovely new husbands (usually other Italian immigrants) for widowed ladies, a benevolent concept if ever there was one. But the reality was anything but benevolent, because shortly after the wedding the unfortunate groom would meet a sudden end and the bride would find herself widowed again—and the beneficiary of her late husband's life insurance policy, thoughtfully arranged by the Petrillo cousins as part of the service. And they, of course, took a generous cut.

ARSENIC INCORPORATED

It wasn't long before the ladies of Philadelphia cottoned on to this cunning concept, and the matrimonial agency became a "murder for hire" organization, because those "sudden ends" were no accident, despite the fact that they were presented as such when it came to claiming the life insurance. Accidental death was subject to "double indemnity"—in other words, double the proceeds. So the Petrillo cousins and their expanding gang of fellow thugs dished out fatal doses of arsenic to their fellow countrymen (later earning the gang the name "Arsenic Incorporated"). Or they sought some other way to be able to profit from the insurance proceeds, such as by drowning their victims, or running them over in cars. As they claimed the insurance, they saw their profits grow. The deprivations of 1930s' Philadelphia held no terrors for the iniquitous Poison Ring.

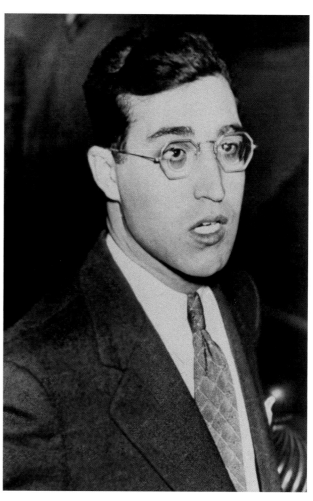

John Cacopardo. *A convict in his own right, he held a grudge against his uncle, Paul Petrillo, and revealed the existence of the Philadelphia Poison Ring in 1936. His lawyer did not believe him and took no action.*

PROFESSIONAL WIDOWS

As the original trio increased to as many as two dozen, even the widows weren't always genuine but members of the gang posing as widows to lure in the hapless bridegrooms. They would come to be known as "professional widows." One of these was Rose Carina, dubbed "Kiss of Death" or "Rose of Death," who lost three husbands in a row at the hands of the murder syndicate. Her first husband was saved by their divorce, but her second husband died in 1931, when the agency was established; her third, in 1933; and her fourth in 1934. Her fifth became a semi-invalid, the result of a stomach ailment.

But this run of deaths went unnoticed by the authorities, despite being impossibly close together, until the plan to murder an Italian laborer named Ferdinand Alfonsi, husband of Stella Alfonsi, finally brought the ring's activities to an abrupt end.

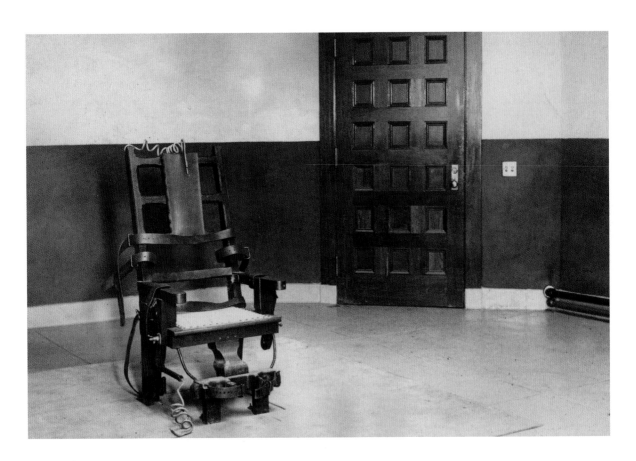

Death sentence. *Electric chairs were given nicknames, including "Old Sparky" and "Old Smokey."*

ENTER THE SNITCH

By late 1938, the increasing number of sudden deaths among the male Italian population of Philadelphia, whose toxicology reports showed higher levels of arsenic than might occur naturally, was starting to attract the attention of the police. And then something happened that made their investigation incredibly simple. An upholstery cleaner named George Myers had run into financial difficulties and approached Herman Petrillo for a loan, whereupon Herman, with an uncharacteristic lack of judgment, offered Myers $600 (or, as an alternative, $2,500 in counterfeit money), to kill Alfonsi, who was proving annoyingly resistant to arsenic poisoning. Herman suggested that Myers should give Alfonsi a hearty whack with a blunt instrument, then pass off his—surely inevitable—demise as an accident.

Myers, however, was not so desperate as to become a murderer, and he reported the conversation to the Philadelphia branch of the Secret Service, which already had Herman in its sights for his counterfeiting activities. An undercover agent approached Herman, who made the same offer, and promptly found his criminal career over.

THE END OF THE ROAD

At this point, everything began to unravel. The trial of Herman Petrillo began on March 13, 1939. An insurance agent saw Herman's photograph in a newspaper and recalled seeing him at the home of Carina Favato—another of the "poison widows"—while he was there to set up life insurance for her stepson, who had subsequently died, as had several other members of her household. The agent informed the police, bodies were exhumed and examined, and the activities of the entire Philadelphia Poison Ring were uncovered.

Trial after trial took place and one after another the ring members were found guilty. In total, the gang was convicted of 70 murders, although it is thought that the tally is nearer 100. Some received commuted death sentences. Ten members, five of whom were women, were sentenced to life imprisonment, and seven others—again including five women—were given prison sentences of up to 20 years. Defended by an exceptionally good advocate and after a very lengthy deliberation, Stella Afonsi was found not guilty of the murder of her husband Ferdinand, who died of arsenic poisoning.

> "I'll let the courts decide whether you were a pawn in the hands of these vicious murders or whether you yourselves were to blame."
>
> *Magistrate Nathan Beifel at the trial of Josephine Romauldo and Agnes Mandiuk*

TAKE A SEAT, MR PETRILLO

As for Herman and Paul, they were eventually convicted of first degree murder in 1941 and executed by electric chair that same year, Paul in the spring and Herman in the fall. Herman protested his innocence to the end and demanded to see the prison governor, but to no avail. The executioner pulled the switch and the activities of the Philadelphia Poison Ring came to an end.

Herman Petrillo's hearing. Had circumstances in the Land of Opportunity been different, would he have lived out his days as a contented spaghetti salesman?

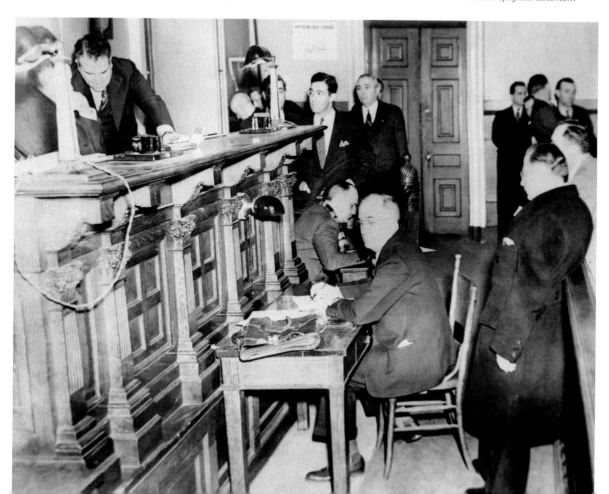

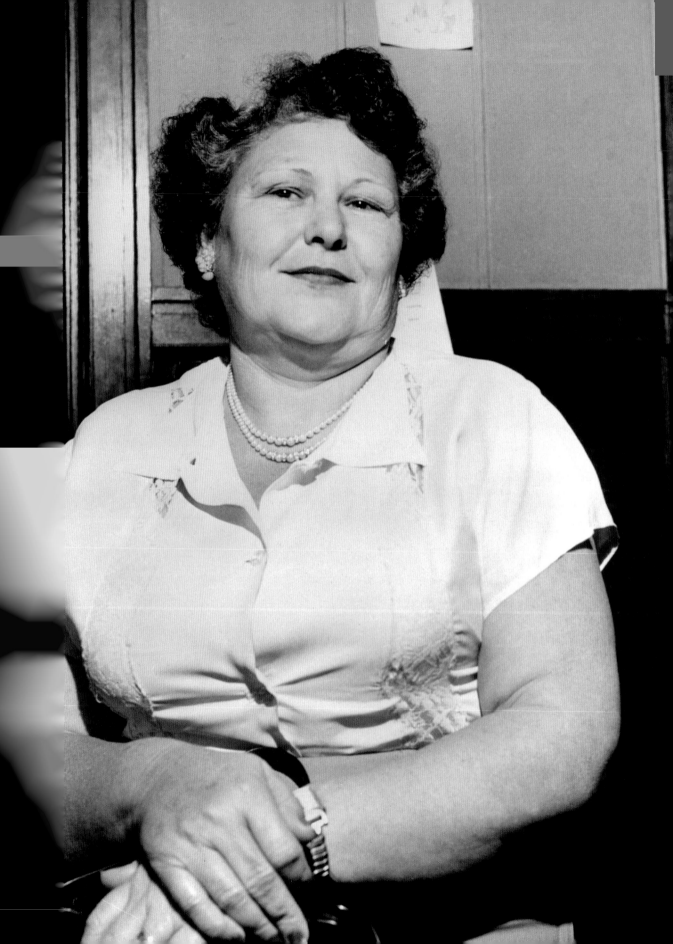

NANNIE DOSS
Laughing all the Way to the Bank

On the surface, Nannie Doss, née Hazle, looked like a character out of a cozy bedtime story. She was plump, with apple cheeks, eyes sparkling through her glasses, and a constant smile. It was hard to believe this comfortable middle-aged lady with her declared enthusiasms for home cooking and true romance magazines could do any harm to anybody.

W HEN NANNIE DOSS WAS ARRESTED on suspicion of the murder of Samuel Doss, her fifth husband, detectives were not prepared for the stream of confessions that was headed their way. And even more disconcerting was the jolly, confiding demeanor of the woman who would shortly earn the label of "the giggling granny" in the press.

A TOUGH UPBRINGING

Information about Nancy Hazle's childhood is sketchy, but it was certainly not easy. She was born in provincial Alabama; Blue Mountain in the early twentieth century was a small settlement, not yet absorbed by the town of Anniston close by. Most people either worked on the land or were employed in the nearby textile mills. Nancy, or Nannie as she was universally known, was the eldest of the five children of James and Lou Hazle. Her father, a farmer, was known locally to be a martinet, very tough on his brood, especially the four girls. He had no hesitation about taking the children out of school if he needed help on the farm, and Nannie's education was neglected. As they grew up, his teenage daughters were not allowed to experiment with pretty clothes or makeup; they were kept at home and not encouraged to socialize at local dances or parties. One childhood incident is on record: at the age of seven years, Nannie was taken on a train to visit relatives in the south of Alabama and took a hard blow to the head when the train stopped suddenly and she hit it on a metal rail. The child was said to have been knocked unconscious, and afterward she always suffered from bad headaches; much later, the accident would be used as evidence to argue that she was mentally unbalanced, or even insane.

"I'm sure I'll find my perfect mate yet." —*Nannie Doss, while being questioned by police about the murder of Samuel Doss*

Mad or bad? *Nannie Doss remained a puzzle to detectives, with her calm manner and her sudden, disconcerting fits of the giggles.*

Although she was unhappy at home, Nannie did have some pleasures. She loved to read romance magazines, leaving behind her comfortless surroundings in fantasies of true love. And she apparently also enjoyed cooking. She was quick to escape to a job at the local linen mill as soon as she was old enough, and it was here that she met the first husband of her long matrimonial career. Of the five men to occupy the role, he would be the only one to die a natural death.

THE ONE THAT GOT AWAY

Nannie was only 16 years old when she married Charlie Braggs in 1921. The young couple had only known each other for a few months but, unusually, her father approved of the match, and her main motive may well have been to escape from home. If so, she soon discovered that she had jumped out of the frying pan into the fire—Charlie lived with his mother and was under her thumb. What was worse, Mrs Braggs senior held many of the same values as Nannie's father—she disapproved of light reading, sitting idly, and having fun. Nevertheless, Nannie and Charlie got on well enough to have four daughters between 1923 and 1927. Each accused the other of infidelity, and the stresses and strains of the marriage resulted in Nannie becoming a heavy drinker and smoker, both habits she kept till the end of her life. Charlie would later tell people that, despite her equable appearance, he had been afraid of her moods.

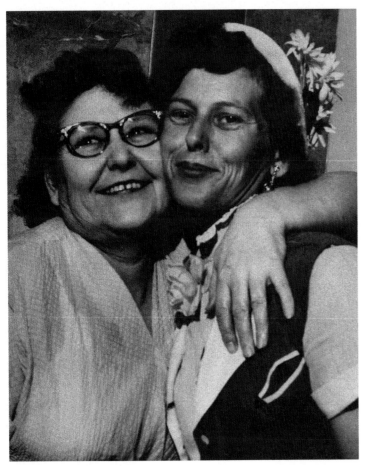

Mother and daughter. *Nannie Doss with her eldest daughter, Melvina, whose second child died shortly after birth.*

In 1927, there was a tragedy. Nannie and Charlie's two middle daughters, both still toddlers, died suddenly, apparently of food poisoning. The family held life insurance policies, so were paid $500 on the death of each child. Shortly afterward, Charlie left home, taking the eldest daughter, Melvina, with him but leaving the youngest, Florine, with Nannie and his mother. He would reappear a year later, having found a new partner, but in the interim his mother died. By 1928, Nannie and Charlie were divorced and Melvina was back living with her mother.

Nannie was at home with her romance magazines once more. But her interest in reading about theoretical love was broadening out into the practical and she turned her attention to a lonely hearts column. It was through an advertisement that she was to meet husband number two, Robert Franklin Harrelson. He was close to her age, 23 to her 24, and after swapping letters and some home baking (Nannie liked to make cakes), the two finally met up. They married in 1929, not very long after her divorce came through and Nannie and her daughters all moved to Jacksonville.

THE LONGEST MARRIAGE

Although the marriage was to last for 16 years, it was a failure almost from the beginning. Harrelson, known as Frank to his friends, was a drunk and would loudly abuse Nannie and the girls when he was in his cups. Still, she seemed to put up with it, and the girls grew up and left home. Melvina married and started a family; her second child died shortly after birth—while still groggy after giving birth, Melvina was reported as saying that she had seen her mother with a hatpin near the baby. No one really believed her; she had only just come round from an anesthetic, and the story just seemed too bizarre. No official investigation of the baby's death was ever made. In 1945, Melvina's first child died while in the care of his grandmother from "unexplained asphyxia." As with her own children, Nannie had insured her grandchild and picked up $500 upon his death.

Nannie and Frank's marriage dragged on unhappily until matters came to a head in August 1945. The end of World War II, with the surrender of Japan, was celebrated heartily in America, and Frank characteristically went out and got very drunk. Nannie claimed that upon his return her husband raped her and two days later, he died. It seems that Nannie had added arsenic to his whiskey. Frank's life had also been insured, and this time Nannie collected $2,000. A pattern was emerging.

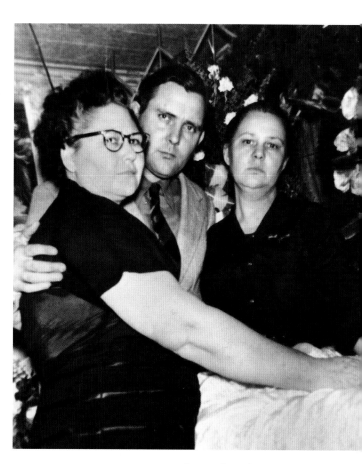

Comforting the widow. *Nannie being supported by friends at the funeral of her third husband, Arlie Lanning, in February 1952.*

His death failed to arouse any suspicions, and Nannie was not on her own for long. Her third husband, Arlie Lanning, was another find from the lonely hearts columns, and the pair decided they were right for each other straight away. They were married within a couple of days of their first meeting, settling down in Lexington, North Carolina. Unfortunately, this search for true love was no more successful than the others; like Frank, Arlie was a heavy drinker. Nannie spent much of their marriage visiting friends and family, however, and the pair were never seen arguing in public. When, after nearly three years of marriage, Arlie became ill and died—apparently suffering from a very bad dose of the flu—Nannie's neighbors were sympathetic. The insurance money, which this time amounted to $1,500, was forthcoming, but shortly after Arlie's death, the family home burned down. Like Arlie, the house had been insured and a check was sent to Nannie for the damages.

"BAD LUCK SEEMED TO FOLLOW HER AROUND"

The lonely hearts columns had not served Nannie particularly well, so for her next foray into romance, she tried a dating group instead, the "Diamond Circle Club." They offered an introduction to her fourth husband, Richard Morton, of Emporia, Kansas, and she married him in 1952. Unlike Frank and Arlie, he was not a drinker, but he was, according to some, a womanizer, and he was frequently away from home. After the death of Nannie's father in early 1953, Nannie's mother came to stay with the couple, but the visit was short-lived; just a few days after her arrival, she collapsed and died, complaining of bad indigestion. Richard followed her three months later, shortly, it seems, after downing a whole flask of Nannie's coffee. It had been a brief marriage but Richard's life insurance brought in another $1,500.

Nannie's fifth and final husband was Samuel Doss. Unlike her previous spouses, Doss was a churchgoing man, a respectable widower from Tulsa, Oklahoma. In theory, he should have been a keeper, but shortly after the two married in June 1953, Nannie began to find life with him irksome. There was so much that he frowned upon. He did not like her reading her romance magazines or listening to the radio, and he would not let her visit with the neighbors and enjoy their new television set. Other women might have chafed against these restrictions, but in imposing them on Nannie, Samuel Doss was signing his own death warrant. By September 1953, he was in hospital with crippling stomach cramps after eating stewed prunes prepared by his wife, and although he recovered briefly and was sent home on October 5, a sudden relapse that evening killed him.

"She was as calm and composed as she might have been if she were being baptized." —*The police stenographer who recorded Nannie's statement*

A MURDERER UNCOVERED

Finally, Nannie had overreached herself. Samuel Doss had had not one but two life insurance policies, and perhaps Nannie had been in too much hurry to collect. Doctors who had been treating Samuel had been pleased by his progress, though, and were puzzled by his sudden death. When they told Nannie that they wanted an autopsy, she agreed that it would be a good idea, and a huge quantity of arsenic was found in the body. On November 26, she was arrested and taken in for questioning.

Detectives were about to undergo one of the most bizarre interviews any of them ever experienced. Nannie sat cheerfully in her chair, at first denying all knowledge of wrongdoing. Gradually, as she was presented with individual snippets from the growing pile of evidence, she began, smilingly, to confess. Every so often she would be challenged on a specific point and would give an eerie little giggle, followed by the sly admission, "I guess I lied about that." Point by point, they wore her down, interviewing in pairs, a new team taking over when one set had had enough. Nannie gradually began sharing information: her husbands had died because they had annoyed her, drunk too much, or gone out womanizing. She presented the poisonings as though they were a sensible option. Samuel had died, she said, "because he got on my nerves."

Was Nannie mad? She told her questioners about the blow to the head she had had as a child and about the headaches she had suffered from ever since. The way she laughed her way through her admissions sounded deranged. The only time she became indignant was when it was suggested that she had murdered blood relatives—although it is highly likely that she was responsible for at least some of the other deaths around her—but she seemed to feel that murdering a husband was one thing, and doing away with a family member quite another. When detectives asked her what punishment she felt she should be given for murdering four husbands and a probable six or seven other people, she smiled and said they should do "whatever they liked" to her.

Eventually, however, Nannie was deemed sane enough to stand trial. Despite her confessions, she was tried for the murder of one husband only: Samuel Doss. She pleaded guilty but continued to laugh and smile in the courtroom through even the most harrowing accounts of his suffering. On May 18, 1955, she was sentenced to life imprisonment for murder, escaping the electric chair. She died of leukemia less than ten years later in a prison hospital ward. Toward the end of her life, she allegedly expressed disappointment with her job at McAlester Prison in Oklahoma, complaining she was confined to working in the laundry. When they were shorthanded, she would offer to help out, but no one would ever allow her a job in the kitchen.

Irrepressibly cheerful. Nannie Doss smiles her way through her confession to murder as she is questioned in detail by Captain Harry Stege.

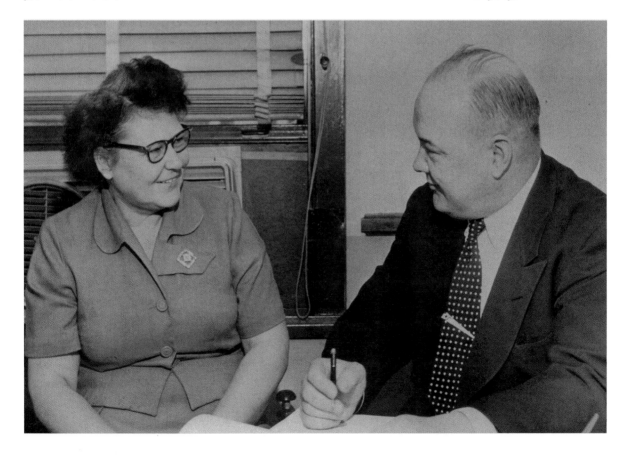

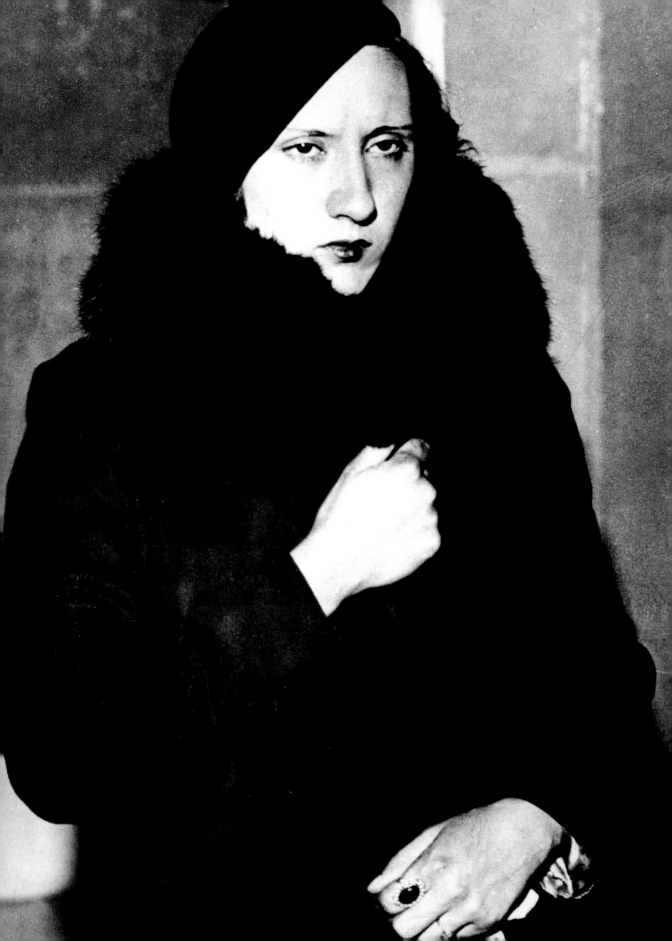

VIOLETTE NOZIÈRE
The Murder that Shocked Paris

Rue de Madagascar was a quiet street in a respectable, largely working-class area of Paris, so the disturbance at number 9 late at night on Monday, August 21, 1933, was unusual. The noisy pounding on an apartment door was followed by hysterical yelling—a girl screaming loudly enough for the whole street to hear. "Monsieur Mayeul," she shouted. "Quickly, quickly—something horrible has happened!"

POISONER

Violette Nozière
Born: January 11, 1915,
  Neuvy sur Loire, France
Died: November 26, 1966,
  Paris, France
Motive: Possibly for financial
  gain, or to take revenge on
  incestuous abuse
Poison: Veronal, a branded
  sleeping mixture
  containing barbiturate
Number of victims: 1

THE GIRL ON THE DOORSTEP of the Mayeuls' sixth-floor apartment was Violette, the 18-year-old daughter of their neighbors, Germaine and Jean-Baptiste Nozière. As Monsieur Mayeul stepped into the hallway, he noticed a strong smell of gas. Rushing into the Nozières' flat across the passage, he ran into the kitchen and turned off the open—though unlit—jets of the range, then flung the windows open. Pressing a towel over his mouth and nose, he went through to the bedroom, where he saw his neighbors, apparently lifeless, lying on the bed. He said later that his immediate impression was of a joint suicide.

By now, the whole house was awake, and someone had gone to telephone for both an ambulance and the police. Number 9 had six floors and was home to 40 families, and the staircase was full of people, discussing what had happened and wondering how. Concerned neighbors ushered Violette, by now gabbling about the money worries her parents had had, out of the flat.

The ambulance had arrived and the medics were just loading the body of Monsieur Nozière onto a stretcher, when one of them noticed a tiny motion from the other figure on the bed. Holding a mirror close to Germaine Nozière's face, he saw a faint mist—she was not quite dead. So while her husband was ferried to the morgue, Madame Nozière was rushed to the local hospital, where the doctors managed to stabilize her, although she was to remain in a coma for some days.

SUICIDE ... OR MURDER?

What could have induced the Nozières to do such a terrible thing? The unwashed dishes on the dining table seemed to show that three people had eaten supper earlier that evening, but Violette said that she had found her parents like that on returning home after a few days staying with friends. Who had dined with them? Police inquiries around the neighbors soon garnered plenty of gossip. Apparently,

Violette Nozière. Parricide and runaway, Violette was to become notorious throughout France. Her slender figure and elegant dress sense were pored over in the gutter press even as her "degenerate" morals and values were deplored.

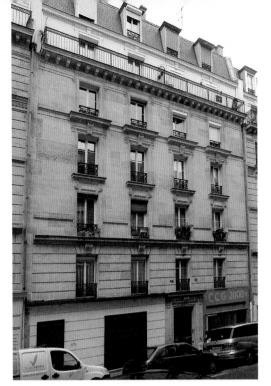

Rue de Madagascar.
Although located in a respectable neighborhood, Rue de Madagascar wasn't a wealthy street—the apartments were small and overcrowded, and everyone knew everyone else's business.

far from being worried about money, the main trouble the Nozières had was with Violette herself. Their only child, she seemed to have gone off the rails a couple of years earlier. She wanted to live independently, she was constantly asking for money, she had numerous boyfriends, she mixed with a louche crowd over on the Left Bank—the rumor mill was hard at work. And while the door-to-door visits were going on, news came from the hospital that what Germaine Nozière was suffering from was not gas poisoning at all, but an overdose of barbiturates. Someone had turned on the gas when she and her husband were already lying unconscious on the bed.

A full search of the Nozières' apartment revealed wineglasses that contained traces of barbiturates, and a prescription packet from a Dr Deron in the wastebasket. The original suicide theory was looking more unlikely, and the police were beginning to be convinced that they were looking at a murder.

By now, the case had been transferred from the local police to the department of the national force entrusted to deal with serious crimes, based on Quai des Orfèvres beside the river Seine. Heading up the inquiry was Inspector Marcel Guillaume, a highly regarded detective and a well-known figure in Paris.

He tracked down the man Violette often stayed with in the Latin Quarter, a young law student called Jean Dabin, who shared more information about the girl. He admitted that Violette often helped him out with money, bankrolling meals and outings. And where did she get the cash? Apparently, it was given to her by older men in return for "dates," but in reality, she was secretly engaged in an amateur form of prostitution.

> "Violette killed her father like a cannibal, because she wanted to eat and drink up the savings that were his French life and blood."
>
> Janet Flanner, *Paris correspondent for* The New Yorker

WHAT REALLY HAPPENED AT RUE DE MADAGASCAR

Violette was sounding less and less like the concerned daughter who had banged on the Mayeuls' front door to get help. She had spent the night of August 21 at the concierge's apartment. On the afternoon of Wednesday August 23, the police took her to visit her mother, who was improving but had not yet regained consciousness. However, she left the hospital without her escort, and disappeared.

The picture that was emerging was completed when Germaine Nozière emerged from her coma and promptly accused Violette of poisoning her and her husband. In Germaine's account, the dishes on the table were from the Sunday, not the Monday night. On August 20, Violette had dined with her parents and, since neither was feeling well, had suggested they take some medicine for headaches that she told them had been prescribed by Dr Deron. She poured the powder into their wine and then, when they went to lie down complaining of feeling even worse, said she would run to consult the doctor. Returning a little later, she claimed that he had recommended taking some baking soda, before giving them another dose of what would turn out to be Veronal, rendering them both unconscious. Most chilling of all, she then pocketed the substantial sum of money that was usually kept hidden away in the apartment and left for a full night and a day, spent shopping and partying with her friends, before returning to turn on the gas, "find" her parents, and raise the alarm.

VIOLETTE'S STORY

In just a few days, Violette Nozière had gone from "person of interest" to "most wanted." Police spoke to everyone she knew, but for a few days there was no trace of her. On August 29, their luck changed. Detectives received a call from a Pierre Gourcerol, a young cavalry officer on leave in Paris, who had made a date for that evening with a pretty girl calling herself Christiane d'Arfeuil. He thought her manner odd, and also that she looked like the by now notorious Violette. Police went to the brasserie where the couple had arranged to meet and arrested Violette when she arrived.

The case had been the front page story in every newspaper for a week. Le Petit Parisien and Le Journal were full of highly colored stories about Violette, the party girl who sold herself to men, the fantasist from a solid, working-class background who had tried to murder her parents for money. She had used some of the cash she had taken from the apartment to buy a chic new outfit—a skirt and sweater, beret, and coat with fur collar, all in fashionable black—so the pictures taken on her arrest supported the image drawn in the popular press of Violette as a glamorous ne'er-do-well.

Inspector Guillaume was the first to interview her, and it was to him that Violette dropped her bombshell. She freely admitted to poisoning her parents, but she told him that she had not intended to kill her mother and had given her less of the poison; her real target was her father, who had been abusing her since she was 12 years old. Were these stories of incest true? In his memoirs, written years later, Guillaume, a shrewd judge of character, was to say that he had believed her. However, it took a year for Violette to come to trial, and by then her image as a scarlet woman had become so entrenched that the judge opened by accusing her of being a habitual liar and a fantasist. Her accusations against her father were dismissed as grossly slanderous and she was found guilty of murder, with the motive of inheriting her parents' savings, and sentenced to execution—commuted soon after to life imprisonment.

She was to serve just 12 years in prison. Freed in 1945, she lived for a further two decades, marrying and giving birth to five children. By the time she died, she was a respectable matron, a devout Christian, loved by her family. Perhaps most surprisingly of all, Germaine Nozière went to live with Violette and her husband, and outlived her notorious daughter by a couple of years.

POISON CABINET

Veronal was not an unusual drug in the 1930s, and it was a common cause of accidental poisonings. It was the first barbiturate available over-the-counter, and could often be bought without a prescription. A moderate dose would work within an hour and produce a sound night's sleep; an overdose, however, could send the taker into a coma from which they might never wake.

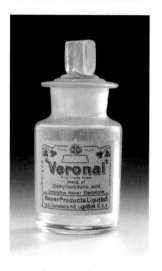

Veronal. *First marketed in 1903, by the 1930s the neat little bottle was a familiar sight in many family medicine cabinets.*

FROM FACT TO FICTION
Inspector Guillaume was the most famous policeman of his time in Paris, and is said to have been an inspiration for Georges Simenon's famous fictional detective, Inspector Maigret. Guillaume and Simenon were close friends, and Guillaume shared many of Maigret's characteristics, known for his calm, phlegmatic, and thorough approach to even the most challenging case—although, unlike Maigret, he preferred cigarettes to a pipe.

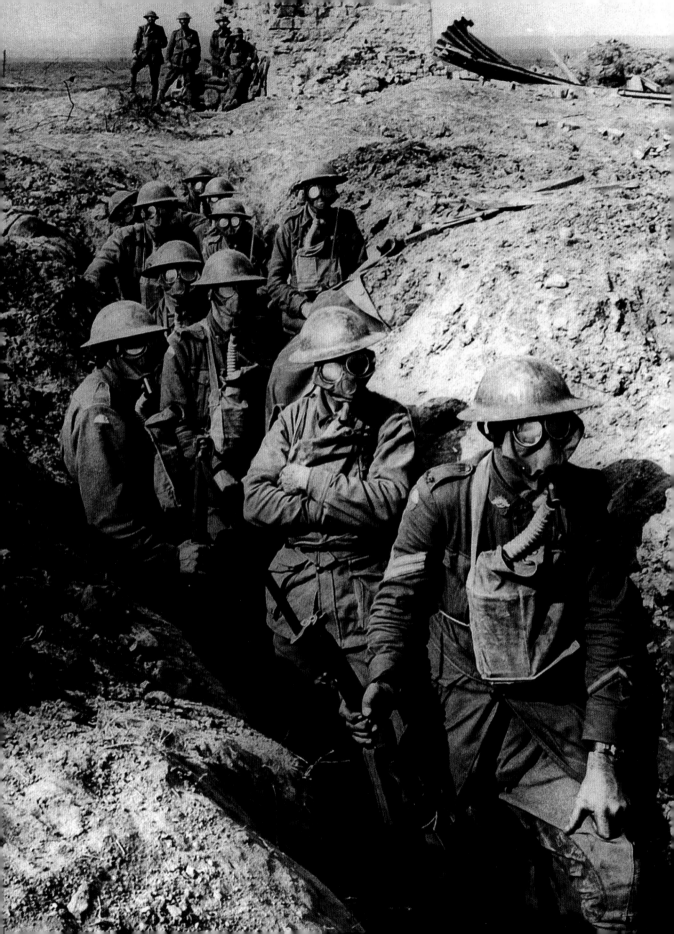

POISONS IN WARFARE
A History of Chemical Weapons

For many hundreds of years, men waged war with physical weapons—swords, crossbows, cannons, bayonets, hand grenades, guns. Tactics played a huge part, but when it came to the hardware, there was no subtlety—those going into battle knew what to expect. But on April 22, 1915, the game changed. Poison gas, silent and often insidious, became the new weapon of war.

IN AUGUST 1914, Germany declared war on Russia and France, Britain declared war on Germany, and Germany invaded France and Belgium. In the early months of the Great War, or World War I, as the conflict would come to be known, there were some unsuccessful skirmishes using gas. The French fired grenades at the Germans containing xylyl bromide, so-called tear gas, which irritates the mucous membranes of the eyes but is rarely permanently disabling; the Germans then fired shells at the British containing dianisidine chlorosulfate, a lung irritant that was destroyed when the shells exploded so had very little effect beyond causing sneezing fits; and in January 1915, the Germans fired howitzer shells at the Russians containing liquid tear gas, which again was rendered completely ineffective, this time because of the freezing winter temperatures at the Eastern Front.

> "A cynical and barbarous disregard of the well-known usages of civilised war."
>
> Sir John French, *Commander of the British Expeditionary Force*

THE GREAT WAR

While the Germans at this stage were concentrating their efforts on the Eastern Front, on April 22, 1915, in an attempt to divert the attention of the British, Canadian, and French Allied forces, they launched an attack on the Ypres Salient, a short stretch of the extensive Western Front, where French and Algerian soldiers were "dug in" in trenches. The attack began with heavy bombardment around the Belgian town of Ypres, but in the early evening sentries along the defensive line noticed a strange yellow-green cloud wafting toward them. They had no way of knowing that the cloud had been created by 400 tons of chlorine gas. Within moments of reaching its victims, the gas tore at their throats, leaving them suffocating and helpless. The enemy were disabling the Allied troops before

Trench warfare. *Gas masks became an essential element of the soldier's uniform after the introduction of pulmonary agents in World War I.*

POISON CABINET

ZYKLON B

Zyklon B was made from pellets of diatomaceous earth, roughly the size of peas, saturated with hydrogen cyanide (chemical formula HCN), also known as prussic acid. Hydrogen cyanide is a volatile, colorless liquid with an odor of bitter almonds. It passes into the bloodstream via the mucus membranes, the skin, and especially through the lungs, where it neutralizes respiratory enzymes and blocks the ability of the body's cells to absorb oxygen. Brain cells can withstand this absence of oxygen, known as anoxia, for only about 15 seconds before the victim becomes unconscious. Asphyxiation, and death, follow within 20 minutes.

they could charge in on horseback, protected by crude gas masks. But the chlorine gas was merely an experiment, and worse was to come. January 1916 saw the unleashing on the Eastern Front of phosgene gas, six times deadlier than chlorine and colorless so that its victims could not detect it by sight, but they would certainly know about its effects within a day or two, when their lungs would fill with fluid, heralding an agonizing death. In 1917, the Germans introduced "mustard" gas, named for its odor, which could penetrate clothing and be absorbed through the skin, causing severe blistering. By the end of World War I, nearly 100,000 people had died from the use of chemical weapons and a million more were left injured; and while gas accounted for only 3 percent of total fatalities, fear alone of being gassed had a hugely detrimental effect on morale.

FRITZ HABER

Poison gas was the brainchild of a German named Fritz Haber, who in 1918 won the Nobel Prize for Chemistry for his work on converting nitrogen to produce an inexpensive fertilizer to enhance agricultural output. However, at the outbreak of World War I, Haber and his team had also begun work on developing gas as a weapon, and while the Allies were outraged at the use of chemical warfare, considering it to be at the very least unchivalrous (the use of asphyxiating gases in war had been prohibited by the 1899 Hague Convention), Haber considered it no worse than killing the enemy with artillery.

As part of his agricultural research, Haber also helped develop pesticide gases, the name of one of which, Zyklon B, would come to be famous, or rather infamous, for its most cruel of uses—to exterminate Jewish prisoners of war in the concentration camps of Nazi Germany. Prior to World War II, Zyklon B was put to

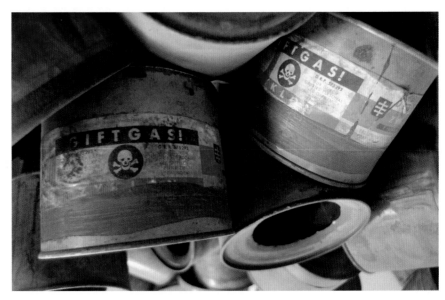

Giftgas! ("*Poison gas*") *warns the label on tins of Zyklon B, the pesticide turned weapon of mass destruction used at Nazi extermination camps during World War II.*

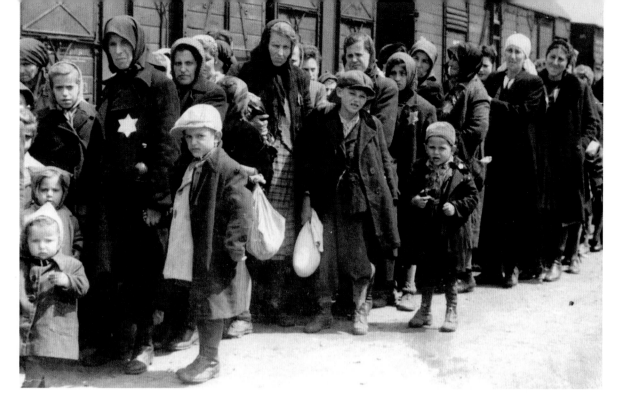

innocent use in Germany to disinfect and exterminate pests. Once the war was underway, it was used in the concentration camp at Auschwitz for sanitation and pest control; however, from August 1941 it took on a new and far more sinister role, at first experimentally and then routinely, for the mass annihilation of prisoners who had been "selected for death." The Zyklon B used at Auschwitz was produced by Degesch (Deutsche Gesellschaft für Schädlingsbekämpfung mbH), the German Corporation for Pest Control. The patent for the pesticide was held by IG Farbenindustrie, a conglomerate of German chemical manufacturers, which contributed generously to the Nazi Party in 1933, despite having several Jewish board members.

Death train. *Women and children arrive at Auschwitz on a deportation train, c.1942. The star-shaped badges sewn on the coats of some of the women identified them as Jews.*

"THE MOST DREADFUL OF HORRORS"

Prisoners who had been selected for death at Auschwitz were told to undress, often in the open air, and were then herded, naked, into the extermination chambers. Once the chambers were full, the doors were shut and the Zyklon B pellets were released into the chamber through vents. Those standing closest to the vents were fortunate, as they died almost immediately; for those further

AN AWFUL IRONY

Fritz Haber was himself a Jew. Once Hitler came to power in 1933 he resigned and, feeling too vulnerable to remain in Germany despite his contribution to the war effort, left the country. He died of a heart attack in January 1934. His wife, who was horrified by her husband's part in the chlorine gas experiment at Ypres in April 1915, had shot herself with Haber's service revolver soon afterward; several members of his extended family, including several nieces and nephews, died in the gas chambers; and his only son committed suicide in 1946.

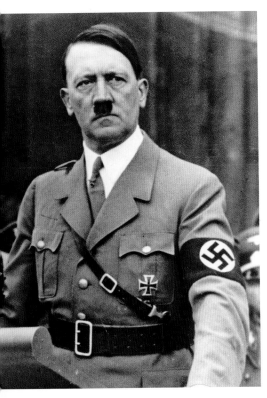

away, death took up to 20 minutes. The chambers were often so overcrowded that the victims had nowhere to fall, and their corpses were found squashed together in the half-squatting position into which they had subsided when the deadly gas overcame them. Their skin was typically discolored pink with red and green spots, and some were found foaming at the mouth, or bleeding from the ears.

Although the victims were told that they had to strip because they were going into the chambers to take showers or to be deloused, they were under no illusions. The Waffen SS physician Johann Paul Kremer, whose diary provides the most famous insider account of the Nazi extermination process, later testified on the gassing of a group of emaciated women: "I concluded from the behavior of these women that they had no doubt what fate awaited them, as they begged and pleaded to the SS men to spare them their lives." Kremer described their gassing in his diary as "the most dreadful of horrors." He later said: "As an anatomist, I have seen a lot of terrible things: I had had a lot of experience with dead bodies, and yet what I saw that day was like nothing I had ever seen before." Another SS officer declared of Auschwitz: "This is the *anus mundi*."

NAZI CONTRA NAZI

While the Nazis will remain forever in the public consciousness for their use of poison gas on the ill-fated Jewish prisoners of war, they also made extensive use of poison on themselves. On July 20, 1944, an abortive attempt was made on Hitler's life by some of his military leaders, including Field Marshal Erwin Rommel. Not wishing Rommel to be exposed as his enemy, Hitler "invited" him to poison himself with a cyanide capsule, which Rommel duly did on October 14. Within seven months, Hitler himself had committed suicide, having concluded that surrender and capture was inevitable.

Adolf Hitler. *One of the most infamous faces in the modern history of the world. Hitler's suicide in April 1945 effectively ended the war in Europe.*

His wife of 40 hours, Eva Braun, was with him when he shot himself; she committed suicide with cyanide. Heinrich Himmler and Hermann Göring also poisoned themselves, while Hitler's propaganda minister, Joseph Goebbels, and his wife, Magda, murdered their six children with cyanide before killing themselves.

"Shouting and screaming of the victims could be heard through the opening and it was clear that they fought for their lives." —*Johann Kremer*

OPERATION RANCH HAND

The Germans' use of chemical agents in warfare was at first considered very unsporting, but it was not long before others involved in conflict were employing poison, although killing the enemy was not necessarily on the agenda. During the Vietnam War (1955–75), the American military sprayed vast quantities of defoliant over Vietnam, Laos, and Cambodia in an operation codenamed "Ranch Hand." The intention was to strip away the vegetation that provided cover for the Vietcong, the communist guerrilla forces backed by the North Vietnamese army, and to deprive them of food. Among the herbicides sprayed from aircraft and trucks was Agent Orange, one of a range of herbicides containing different chemical additives and all identified by a color— Orange, Pink, Green, Purple, White, and Blue. Agent Orange, the herbicide most widely used in the operation (around 11.4 million US gallons/43.2 million liters), contained a high concentration of the deadly toxin dioxin (see page 11).

Unfortunately, the herbicides were indiscriminate in their action and caused huge problems for the local populations not involved in the fighting, destroying their crops and polluting water sources. Even worse were the long-lasting effects on the health of both the local people and of American war veterans, which are still manifesting today in the form of cancer (in particular of the lymphatic system), birth defects, and severe psychological and neurological problems, among other diseases. It is estimated that around 400,000 people have died or were maimed as a result of Agent Orange poisoning, and that as many as half a million children were born with serious birth defects.

THE AUSCHWITZ DEATH TALLY
Johann Kremer noted in one diary entry that around 1,600 people had been murdered on one day alone; it is estimated that, in total, more than a million Jews were killed at Auschwitz. Despite his obvious distaste for his task, Kremer was found guilty of war crimes at the Auschwitz trial held in November–December 1947, based on the contents of his diaries and having admitted to participating in gassings on 14 occasions during his brief time at the camp, between August 30 and November 18, 1942. He was sentenced to death but the sentence was later commuted to life imprisonment. He was released in 1958 and died in 1965.

LEGISLATION

In 1972, the Biological and Toxin Weapons Convention, the first ever multilateral disarmament treaty banning a comprehensive category of weapons, opened for signature. Although parties to the Convention, which came into force in 1975, undertook not to develop, produce, obtain, or stockpile chemical agents for use in warfare, there was no mechanism to ensure compliance. It was updated in 1993 when the Chemical Weapons Convention was signed, coming into force in 1997. Again, the agreement banned the development, production, stockpiling, and use of chemical weapons, but this time with the stipulation that member states of the Organisation for the Prohibition of Chemical Weapons (OPCW) must take the necessary steps to enforce the prohibition. Among the nerve agents banned was one whose name has become all too familiar in recent years: sarin.

Agent Orange. A *specially adapted American military transport aircraft flies low over Vietnam's Mekong Delta, spraying chemical defoliants.*

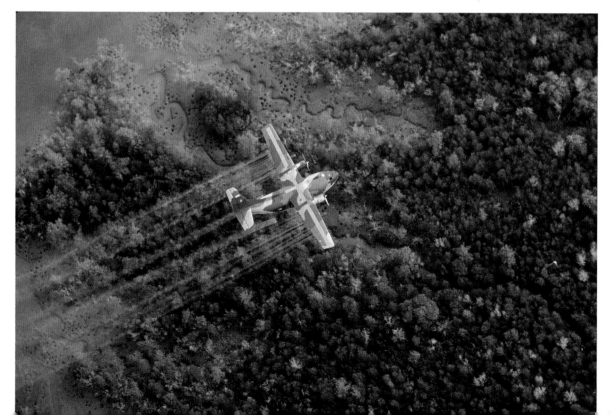

SARIN

Sarin, a clear, colorless, odorless, and tasteless organophosphate, was developed in Germany in 1938 as a pesticide. The Germany army recognized its potential as a weapon and began to manufacture and stockpile it, loaded into shells, although unaccountably it was never used on Allied forces in World War II. In the early years of the Cold War, other countries experimented with sarin, an exercise that served to highlight its dangers. One of its inventors, Otto Ambros, became a consultant on the chemical weapons program in the USA, where a military accident in 1952, involving sarin-filled tanks that fell from an aircraft, resulted in the near death of the one member of the inspection crew not wearing a gas mask. In an even darker incident the following year, a young RAF engineer at the UK's Ministry of Defence laboratory died after taking part in an experiment carried out in a sealed gas chamber, in which liquid sarin was dripped on his arm.

SARIN IN SYRIA

The Chemical Weapons Convention was tested in 2013, when the Syrian military unleashed sarin gas on civilians during the Syrian Civil War, which had begun with anti-government protests in March 2011 and escalated into a full-scale conflict as rebel brigades battled government forces for control of the country, including the capital, Damascus, and the second city, Aleppo. The sarin attack took place in August 2013, when rockets filled with the nerve agent were fired at several suburbs of Damascus, killing about 1,300 people. The threat of US military intervention halted further attacks for a time, and the Syrian president, Bashar al-Assad, agreed to the removal and destruction of the country's entire chemical weapons arsenal. Syria entered the OPCW in October 2013 and the operation to dispose of the arsenal was completed in 2014, although the use of toxic chemicals continued in the meantime, with reports of chlorine being unleashed on rebel-held areas between April and June of that year. In April 2017, a further sarin attack was made, this time on the rebel-held town of Khan Shaykhun.

Halabja cemetery. A solitary figure wanders among the orderly rows of mass graves at Halabja, where the victims of Saddam Hussein's 1988 massacre are laid to rest.

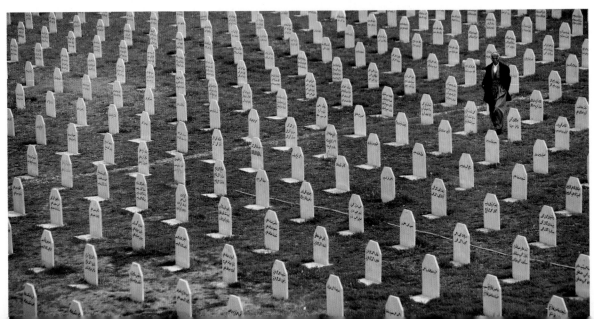

TIMELINE: CHEMICAL WARFARE

600 BCE	Athenian military use poisonous hellebore plants to poison the water supply of the besieged city of Kirrha during the First Sacred War.
429 BCE	Peloponnesian army uses sulfur fumes against the town of Plataea.
1675	France and Germany sign the Strasbourg Agreement, the first international agreement to ban chemical warfare (poison-laced bullets).
1861–65	Proposals for weapons not executed during the American Civil War include the use of cayenne pepper, snuff, chloroform, chlorine, hydrogen cyanide, arsenic compounds, sulfur, and acid, usually in the form of explosive artillery projectiles or poison gas balloons.
1874–1907	International treaties signed by most Western nations to ban the use of poison and poisonous weapons in warfare.
1914–18	First use of chemicals as weapons of mass destruction. French deploy tear gas, Germans deploy chlorine gas at Ypres and use mustard gas, British release chlorine gas from cylinders against Germans at Battle of Loos. Phosgene first used in battle by Germans and then by the Allies. Over a million casualties caused by chemical warfare, mostly by phosgene.
1925	Geneva Protocol bans the use of chemical and biological agents in war but not their development or stockpiling.
1935–36	Benito Mussolini drops mustard gas in Ethiopia to destroy Emperor Haile Selassie's army.
1936	German chemist Gerhard Schrader synthesizes tabun, a potent nerve poison, as a pesticide.
1938	Sarin gas synthesized in Germany.
1939–45	Poison gases used by the Nazis in concentration camps during World War II and by the Japanese army in Asia. Chemicals are not used on European battlefields.
1953	British serviceman Ronald Maddison exposed to sarin during a medical experiment at a Ministry of Defence laboratory.
1961–71	Agent Orange and napalm used by the United States during the Vietnam War.
1972	Biological and Toxin Weapons Convention bans possession and development of biological weapons.
1988	Sarin (and tabun and VX) gas attack on Kurds by Iraq under Saddam Hussein.
1993	Chemical Weapons Convention signed, banning development, production, stockpiling, and use of chemical weapons.
2013	Syrian military uses sarin gas against civilians in Syrian Civil War. Syrian-declared arsenal of chemical weapons neutralized by US military and civilian experts.
2014–15	Chlorine attacks by Syrian regime and mustard gas attack by IS group.
2017	Sarin used in an attack in Syrian town of Khan Shaykhun.
2018	Plan launched by the United States and 28 other countries to identify and punish users of chemical weapons. Suspected chlorine gas/sarin attack in Syrian town of Douma.

POISONS

Chlorine gas: Irritates the eyes, nose, lungs, and throat and provokes choking fits.

Phosgene: Six times more deadly than chlorine gas; causes suffocation.

Mustard gas: Causes temporary blindness, severe blisters on and in the body, attacks lung tissue.

Sarin (GB): Nerve agent that reacts on contact with the skin or when inhaled; attacks the nervous and muscular system.

VX: Most powerful of all nerve agents (100 times more deadly than sarin); capable of killing within minutes of being inhaled by causing fatal disruption of the nervous system. Declared a weapon of mass destruction by the UN.

Tabun (GA): Toxic even when in minute doses; tabun attacks the nervous and muscular system.

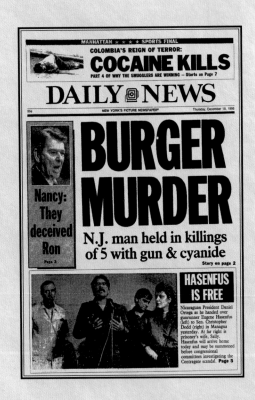

MANHATTAN ★ ★ ★ ★ SPORTS FINAL

COLOMBIA'S REIGN OF TERROR:

COCAINE KILLS

PART 4 OF WHY THE SMUGGLERS ARE WINNING — Starts on Page 7

DAILY ◉ NEWS

35¢   NEW YORK'S PICTURE NEWSPAPER®   Thursday, December 18, 1986

Nancy: They deceived Ron
Page 3

BURGER MURDER

N.J. man held in killings of 5 with gun & cyanide
Story on page 2

HASENFUS IS FREE

Nicaraguan President Daniel Ortega as he handed over gunrunner Eugene Hasenfus (left) to Sen. Christopher Dodd (right) in Managua yesterday. At far right is prisoner's wife, Sally. Hasenfus will arrive home today and may be summoned before congressional committees investigating the Contragate scandal. **Page 5**

CHAPTER FIVE

FROM CULTS TO CONTEMPORARY ESPIONAGE

The art of poisoning has changed with the times, in terms of both the poison itself and the way that it is applied. Sarin—used to murder indiscriminately in the Tokyo subway—and dioxin—which disfigured Ukrainian president Viktor Yuschenko—are both byproducts of modern herbicides and pesticides. The Reverend Jim Jones induced over 900 people to self-administer cyanide laced with tranquilizers, and the twentieth century saw the first splitting of the atom, which would eventually lead to the polonium that killed Russian agent Vladimir Litvinenko. Two twentieth-century poisoners bucked the trend, however—English physician Harold Shipman with morphine, first isolated as an analgesic in 1804, and contract killer Richard Kuklinski, who used cyanide as part of his murder toolkit— the passage of time had not diminished their efficacy.

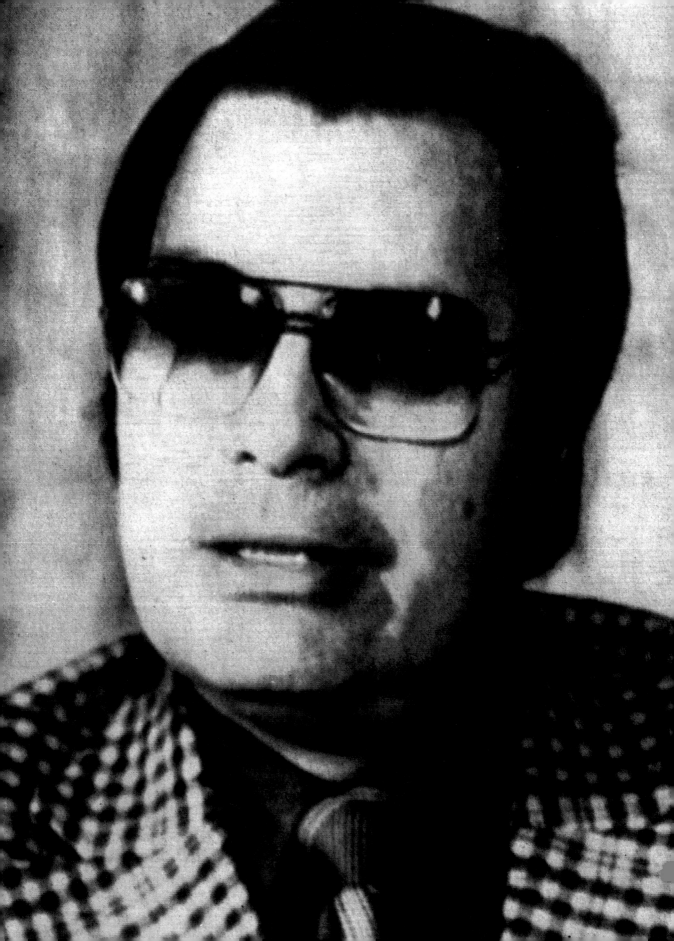

THE REV JIM JONES
Massacre in the Jungle

It was supposed to be a new, idealistic society, set deep in the South American jungle, whose members would live happily together, everyone valued equally, whatever their background, education, or color. So how did this small Utopia end in such carnage, with 918 residents lying dead in the mud? Forty years on, the Jonestown massacre stands out as one of the bloodiest tragedies in American history.

POISONER

James Warren "Jim" Jones
Born: May 13, 1931, Crete, Indiana, USA
Died: November 18, 1978, Jonestown, Guyana, South America
Motive: Mass "revolutionary suicide"
Poison: Cyanide, valium
Number of victims: 918

JAMES JONES, now notorious all over the world for the coercive murder of his flock, was born in a small town in Indiana. His father, James Jones Senior, a disabled veteran of World War I and a member of the Ku Klux Klan, has been described variously as uninterested in him or actively abusive, and the young Jim seems to have begun attending church at the behest of concerned neighbors. He quickly acquired religious zeal of his own, and is said to have begun preaching at the age of ten, loving the prestige and the influence over others that it gave him.

Jim's parents separated in his teens and his mother Lynetta moved to Richmond, Indiana, taking her son with her. He graduated from high school at the end of 1948, and began to study at Indiana University. He also worked shifts as a medical orderly, and it was at the hospital that he met Marceline Baldwin, a student nurse whom he was to marry in 1949. In 1952, he made his first full step toward a future in the church when he was appointed as a student pastor at the Somerset Methodist Church in Indianapolis. Within three years he had founded his own church, first named the Wings of Deliverance but which soon became known as the Peoples Temple. It fast gained a reputation for inclusiveness in an era when congregations were rarely integrated—Jones welcomed everyone, black, white, rich, and poor, to worship with him. His political interests were as strong as his religious ones, and he claimed to be a committed Marxist alongside his other beliefs. At a time when racism was deeply embedded in the southern states, he was a firm advocate for civil rights, attending rallies and protests. He practiced what he preached, too: he and Marceline were possibly the first adopters—literally—of the idea of a "rainbow family," with a growing brood of adoptive children of different ethnicities.

Back in church, his style was vividly evangelical and he was keen on showy demonstrations of the power of faith; in particular, he became enthusiastic about healing services, asserting that he could cure everything from epilepsy to cancer.

The Reverend Jim Jones. *Pictured during the Redwood Valley years, Jim wore dark glasses almost constantly. The loud, checked sport coat and colored shirt and tie are also characteristically flamboyant.*

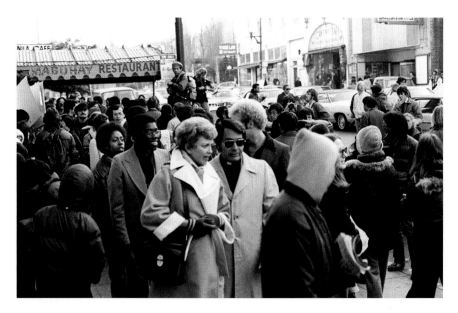

Man of the people. Jones attending a protest against evictions in San Francisco. In the course of the 1960s, he became well-known for supporting the rights of minorities, the poor, and uneducated—those who he felt did not have a voice in society.

He would sometimes claim to have pulled the cancer out of worshipers' bodies, waving handfuls of chickens' guts to "prove" the cure.

By his mid-20s, Jones was an odd mixture of political activist, charismatic young pastor, and charlatan. Instantly recognizable with his pale face, floppy dark hair, and the dark glasses he often wore, he was widely admired as a force for the good—an attractive, dynamic young churchman who could get things done. Critics disliked his showy style and noted a manipulative streak in his dealings with his parishioners, along with an attitude that declared that anyone who was not with him was against him. He called himself "Father" and worshipers were variously his "children" or his "darlings." One thing was certain: most followed his orders without question. What Jim Jones said went.

THE MOVE TO CALIFORNIA

In the early 1960s, Jim Jones started looking at how he could move his church away from Indiana. In 1961, he claimed to have had a dream presaging a nuclear holocaust, and during various trips in the years that followed he sought a new permanent location that would be safer—at least in his view. He considered Cuba and looked at various sites in South America, but eventually fixed on California. In 1965, he transplanted the church and around 150 followers to Redwood Valley in Mendocino County. He used their new home as a base from which to hold services and launch recruitment drives in both San Francisco and Los Angeles, shipping groups of believers to and from the cities in a fleet of buses. By the early 1970s, membership of the Peoples Temple had risen steeply to somewhere between 3,000 and 5,000 people. The Californian years saw Jones himself gain some powerful admirers—and an equal number of critics. While his enthusiasm for rescuing the troubled and underprivileged won plaudits from local politicians and gave him influence with congressmen and councils, his methods were beginning to be subjected to much closer examination, although attempts to run a seven-part exposé in the *San Francisco Examiner* in 1972 were largely thwarted after only three parts had been published, when Peoples Temple members held a vigil outside the newspaper's offices.

It was also difficult to leave the church. Members who decided to go were branded "traitors" and "defectors," and their friends on the outside observed that they seemed genuinely frightened of the consequences of leaving. Reports were being circulated that Jones's original mistrustfulness toward outsiders was becoming outright paranoia. Perhaps most worrying of all, there were quieter murmurings that "Father," who had always been able to preach for hours without flagging, was also taking high quantities of drugs to manage his punishing self-inflicted schedules. The original picture of an inclusive, cooperative, and socially idealistic community was falling apart.

A NEW EDEN

The move to California had proved successful in terms of gaining followers for the Temple, but Jones's ultimate aim was still to center his operations somewhere much more remote. In 1974, he leased nearly 4,000 acres of land from the government of Guyana, a small, poor country on the northwest tip of South America. Located deep in the jungle, the new base, officially named the Peoples Temple Agricultural Project, but soon to be universally referred to as Jonestown, had the advantage of isolation—and not much else. Its members were not afraid of hard work. Over the first three years there, around a thousand followers who gradually relocated to Guyana built a small town, with houses, a health clinic, and a school for the many young children of the commune.

The new location should also have been reassuring for Jones. His followers were now free of much of the outside influence he feared—Jonestown was so remote that it was difficult to visit. Provided they remained compliant, Jones could run things as he wished. By this time, however, his drug habit was acute, and his paranoia was rising to dangerous levels (after his death, a postmortem would reveal that his daily drug intake would have killed anyone who was not habituated to it). In his distorted view, the world outside Jonestown had become the enemy, and the only safety was within the community itself.

> "He said he was Gandhi, Buddha, Lenin—he said he was the coming back of anybody you'd ever want to come back."
>
> *Teri Buford O'Shea, who left Jonestown three weeks before the suicides*

The site of Jones's Utopia. *Jonestown was located deep in the Guyanan forest, and was notoriously difficult to access—giving Reverend Jones almost complete control over his flock.*

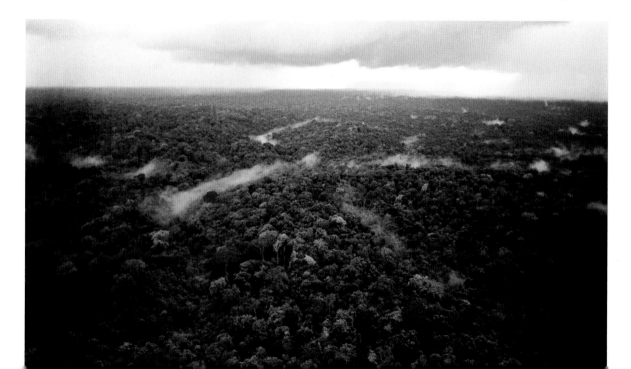

POISON CABINET

Jones killed his followers with a potent mix of cyanide and sedatives stirred up in barrels with a soft drink mix (not actually Kool-Aid, as legend had it, but Flavor Aid). It would have killed them within minutes. He had been stockpiling cyanide for at least two years, having obtained a jeweler's license for it in 1976. Cyanide can be used to clean gold, and, once licensed, the Peoples Temple could order around 1kg/2lb every few months. There is some evidence that he had experimented with its effectiveness; one communication written by a doctor at Jonestown reassured him that "Just two grams is enough to kill a large pig."

"WHITE NIGHTS" IN JONESTOWN

The small number of members who did emerge from Jonestown between late 1975 and 1978 had increasingly worrying news for friends and relatives in the world outside. They told stories of exhausted residents working constantly, seven days a week, of having to listen to hours of Jones's ranting lectures broadcast over loudspeakers, and of armed guards patrolling the borders of the settlement. Most alarming of all was the story of so-called "White Nights" events—suicide drills in which Jones lined up everyone in the settlement and ordered them to drink "poison." "You'll be dead in 40 minutes," he told them, only to reveal, after most had obediently downed their cups, that he was simply carrying out a loyalty test to see who would follow him to the bitter end. Many followers, their families believed, were tired and demoralized; unwilling hostages, they would welcome the opportunity to escape.

The mounting rumors about Jonestown began to attract attention in the American media. By late 1978, one Californian congressman, Leo J Ryan, had heard so many allegations from worried relatives that people were not free to leave the Peoples Temple that he decided to pay a personal visit to Jones and to invite anyone who wanted to leave to return with his party to the United States.

THE FINAL DAY

On November 18, Ryan's plane touched down on the airstrip in Port Kaituma, Guyana. He had come with a television crew and journalists, and initially his group was formally welcomed by Jones, who gave the visitors a tour of Jonestown and spent some time talking to them. They noticed that Jones seemed high, and that he was taking pills constantly, with no break in his continuous harangue about the persecution and lies that were threatening the little Eden he had built in the jungle. When the congressman made it known that anyone who wished to leave could go with him, under his protection, around 20 members came forward, and the group set off back to the airstrip. However, no sooner had they reached it than gunmen from Jonestown who had followed them staged an ambush and opened fire. Congressman Ryan, three members of the press corps, and one of the defectors were killed.

Back at Jonestown, Jones and his inner circle were preparing to die. Followers were summoned to the pavilion, the usual meeting place for Temple members, by loudspeaker announcements. When they arrived, Jones told the assembled group that the time had come for them to join him in what he called "revolutionary suicide." Vats of fruit drink had already been mixed, laced with cyanide and valium. Most seem to have drunk willingly; parents syringed it into their children's mouths, then gulped it down and died on the spot. But a few bodies were found with gunshot wounds; Jones himself died

"They had a choice between being seen as traitors and surviving or drinking the Kool-Aid and being loyal to the cause."

Rebecca Moore, who lost two sisters and a nephew at Jonestown

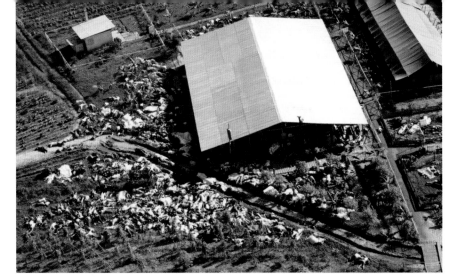

The aftermath of the massacre. *The Guyanese authorities arrived to find a horrendous scene. Jones's followers lay where they had fallen, often embracing one another, with the debris of the poisoning—cups, bottles, and plastic vessels—scattered around them.*

from a shot to the head, probably as a suicide. It was the largest single-event loss of American life before 9/11: 918 people are believed to have died at Jonestown that day, 246 of them children. There were only a handful of survivors; a few had walked into the jungle; one small boy was found hiding a few hundred yards from the compound by the Guyanese police when they arrived at the site next day, and a lady in her 80s, who had been feeling unwell, slept through everything and only awoke when everyone else was dead.

The news stunned the outside world, leaving thousands of bereaved relatives numb. Even those who had thought that Jones was a charlatan and his followers duped cultists found it hard to believe that so many people would be prepared to kill their children and die themselves. They wondered what power he could have had over them. Those who had direct experience of Jim Jones, though, were less surprised. Teri Buford O'Shea, who had joined the Peoples Temple in its Californian days, and who escaped from Jonestown a few weeks before the massacre, said that Jones could deliver whatever a follower was looking for, from religion to socialism. She wrote a book about her experiences and explained, "If you were looking for a father figure, he'd be your father. He always homed in on what you needed and managed to bring you in emotionally."

And if he told you that you must die, apparently you would do that, too.

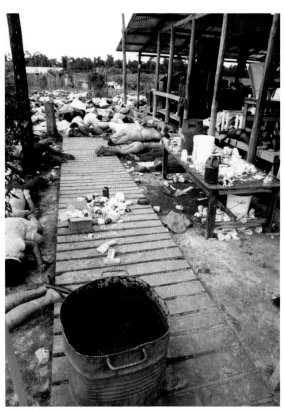

THE DEATH TAPE

A few days after the suicides, investigators found a tape at Jonestown. It was over 44 minutes long and made for harrowing listening. Voices of still-alive commune members could be heard crying and shouting over the moans and screams of the dying. One long-term follower, Christine Miller, was heard trying to stop the carnage, arguing that members could escape to the Soviet Union. Over them, Jones could be heard shouting, "Don't fear death! It is nothing—let's end this now!"

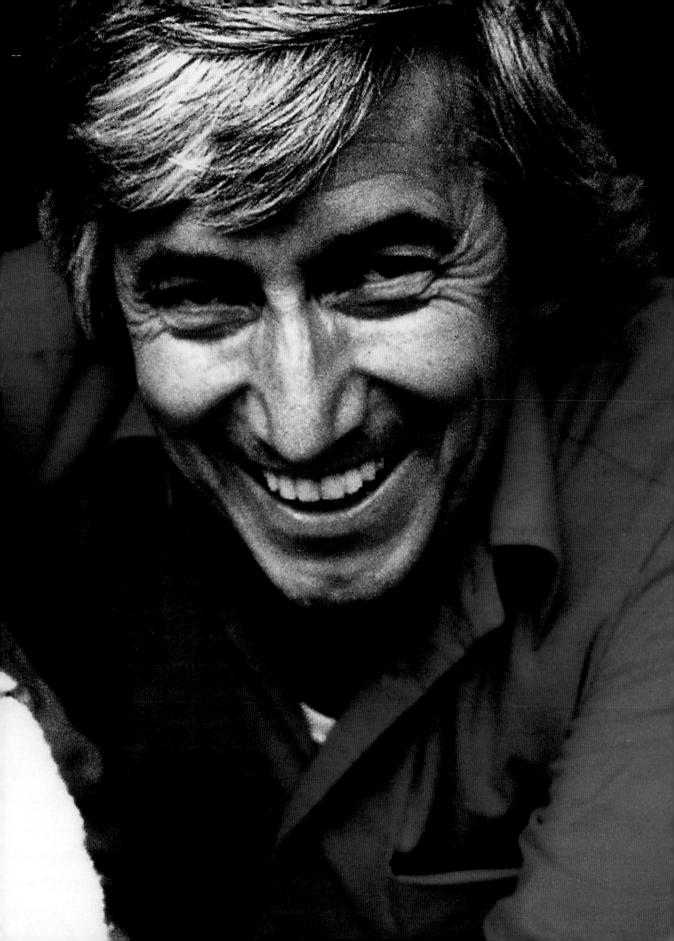

GEORGI MARKOV
The Case of the Poisoned Umbrella

Even in a spy novel it would have been dismissed as far-fetched. A dissident from the Eastern bloc accosted by a mysterious stranger on Waterloo Bridge in the heart of London, then fatally stabbed with a poisoned umbrella—with suspicion falling later on a mysterious attacker named "Agent Piccadilly." But that's apparently exactly what happened in the tragic real-life story of Georgi Markov.

MARKOV WAS BULGARIAN, and had worked as a successful journalist and playwright in his home country. However, his open questioning of Bulgaria's Communist regime had attracted the disapproval of the head of state, Todor Zhivkov. In search of a freer life, Markov defected in 1969 during a visit to his brother, who lived in Italy, then moved to London, where he lived for several years until the time of his death, working as a journalist for the BBC World Service. From 1975, he also made regular broadcasts on Sunday nights for Radio Free Europe, which served countries deemed not to have a free flow of information, and his programs were popular in Bulgaria, reinforcing his role as a thorn in the side of the Communist government.

"I'M SORRY"

Dissidents from Communist countries regularly received death threats in the 1970s and Markov was no exception. In the Bulgarian secret service, Markov had a codename "The Wanderer" and he was certainly a target. Records uncovered after the end of the Cold War and the fall of Communism in Bulgaria suggested that several plans to silence him had already been conceived before the final attack that ended his life.

On the rainy morning of September 7, 1978, Markov was waiting at a bus stop on Waterloo Bridge on his way in to work when he suddenly felt a small, sharp pain in the back of his leg; "It was like an insect bite," he would say later that day. Clapping his hand to the spot, he turned smartly to see a man picking up an umbrella just behind him. "I'm sorry," the man muttered, then quickly crossed the road, hailed a taxi, and was driven off. Markov didn't think anything more of it. He continued on his journey to work, but by the evening he was running a very high fever—high enough for him to be admitted to St James'

Popular journalist. Before defecting during a visit to the West in 1969, Georgi Markov was a popular but contentious journalist and playwright in his native Sofia.

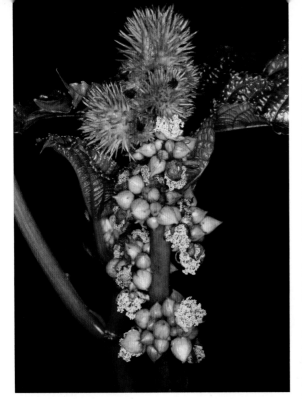

Ricinus communis, *the castor bean or castor oil plant. The lethal dose for adults is considered to be between four and eight beans, but the poison can be extracted in a more concentrated form.*

Hospital in Balham, south London. And at this point he remembered the strange little incident on Waterloo Bridge.

Doctors examined the spot where he'd felt the original pain and, under the surface of the skin, uncovered a tiny metal sphere about the size of the head of a pin. They quickly concluded that he had been poisoned but failed to bring down his fever. In the grip of a raging infection, Markov's body was not strong enough to support him and after three days of excruciating pain, and still running a very high temperature, he died.

FINDING PROOF

The press were hot on the scent of the Markov case. Even before his death, the British newspapers were running lurid headlines about James Bond-style murder weapons. Careful examination of the minute metal sphere revealed that it held an L-shaped compartment with two holes that had originally been sealed with a waxy or sugary substance. It was passed to Porton Down, the top-secret British research and weapons base, where further study concluded that the umbrella Markov had seen had acted as an improvised gun that had introduced the pellet under his skin. His body temperature had melted the sealant, releasing the poison that had killed him. The British public was incredulous: surely someone couldn't be murdered in broad daylight in a highly public place by a secret but highly toxic micro-bullet? The story was just too bizarre and fantastical to be true. That this was exactly what had happened took a little time to sink in. Even Markov's newly bereaved wife found it hard to accept.

"I've been brought up in this country—I can't believe people go round stabbing other people with umbrellas." —Annabel Markov, *upon being told the cause of her husband's sudden illness*

WHO KILLED GEORGI MARKOV?

Both the press and public swiftly came to the same conclusion as the British government—the indications were that Markov had been murdered by the Bulgarian secret services. This view was reinforced by the revelation that another Bulgarian dissident, Vladimir Kostov, who was living in Paris at the time, had experienced an identical attack carried out in his local subway station just ten days before the assault on Markov. Kostov, who had been standing on a subway escalator, said that he had felt a sudden pain, which he compared to a bee sting and this time in his back, but he had been luckier. The tiny pellet had apparently failed to lodge securely under his skin, so he absorbed less of the poison, and although he ran a very high fever for a few days, he survived.

Kostov hadn't seen an umbrella in the course of his attack; he said his attacker was carrying only a briefcase, and this lead to some fresh theories. These included the suggestion that the umbrella Markov had seen was simply a distracting prop, and that he had actually been stabbed by a smaller weapon that would have been easier to aim accurately, perhaps a modified fountain pen.

REVELATIONS

The Communist government in Bulgaria collapsed in 1989 as part of the overall dissolution of the Eastern bloc, and free elections were held the following year. Like other formerly socialist countries, Bulgaria began to examine its past and the murder of Markov came under review. Both journalists and state investigators looked through the previously secret files of the regime and found that the most likely assassin was the so-called "Agent Piccadilly," who was believed to have been Francesco Gullino, born in Italy of Danish parents, a former drug dealer who had been in the pay of the Communist regime for over a decade.

Markov's killing is now believed to have been on the orders of the Darzhavna Sigurnost, the Bulgarian secret services. The story may come closer to the absurd than many spy tales—but there was nothing humorous about the outcome for Georgi Markov.

WHICH POISON?

That the poison used on Markov was ricin went unquestioned for over 20 years, especially after a pig weighing about the same as an adult human died when it was dosed with an equivalent amount of ricin in an experiment at Porton Down. A twenty-first-century reexamination made ricin seem a less certain conclusion; the cavity inside the pellet was re-evaluated and it was found that it would only hold 0.20 of a milligram. Ricin is highly toxic, but the fatal dose for a human is accepted to be closer to 1.7 milligrams. So if the poison wasn't ricin, what was it?

There were several candidates including abrin, another natural poison found in the seeds of *Abrus precatorius*, or the rosary pea, which has similar properties to ricin and yet is substantially stronger. Another potential contender put forward was plutonium. Yet neither was ever proved conclusively.

Could any parallels be drawn with the murder of former KGB officer Alexander Litvinenko (see page 178), who died in London in 2006 after being poisoned with radioactive polonium-210? A number of questions still remain unanswered.

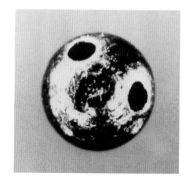

Poison pellet. *The size of a pin head, with a hollow chamber to hold poison, the minute metal pellet that killed Georgi Markov was actually a tiny watch bearing, modified for a much less innocent purpose.*

In memoriam. *People attend a commemoration service in Sofia on September 11, 2013, marking 35 years since the death of Georgi Markov.*

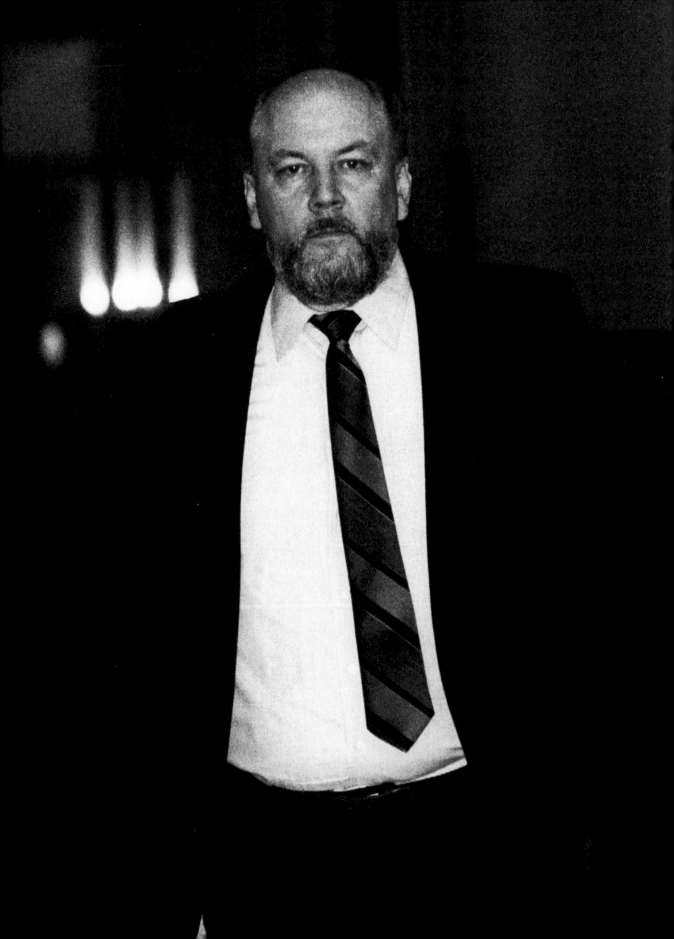

RICHARD KUKLINKSI
"The Ice Man"

In Richard Kuklinski, New York's notorious Mafia families found the perfect hitman, for only the most cold-blooded of killers would take pleasure in spraying cyanide into a victim's face, or freezing a body to obscure the time of death. On the face of it, Kuklinksi was a model citizen. In reality, he was The Ice Man.

POISONER

Richard Leonard Kuklinski
Born: April 11, 1935, Jersey City, New Jersey, USA
Died: March 5, 2006, Trenton, New Jersey, USA
Motive: Murder
Poison: Cyanide (among others)
Number of victims: Convicted of 6 killings, but possibly killed 200+

SOME ARE BORN murderers, and some have murder thrust upon them. It might be argued that Richard Kuklinski had murder thrust upon him as a result of his upbringing—like father, like son, it is said, and Kuklinski's father was of a violent disposition. But as he hit his savage stride and the tally of his victims soared, it became obvious even to Kuklinski that he was a natural-born killer. He felt empowered by killing. He was not a man to cross.

THE MAFIA COMES TO NEW YORK

The New York Mafia learned its craft on the island of Sicily, at that time part of Italy, in the second half of the nineteenth century. The last vestiges of the Italian feudal system were abolished with the country's unification in 1860, and banditry descended upon Sicily as land previously belonging to the nobility was divided among the peasants. The nascent Mafia offered protection to the new landowners and merchants in return for "tribute"—a euphemism for payment—and the protection racket was born. It was effectively a police force that was more corrupt than any criminal.

When Italian immigrants began to flood into America toward the end of the century, members of the Sicilian Mafia were among their number. They continued to offer "protection" to the immigrants and those who declined found themselves in big trouble. For years, the various Mafia gangs jostled for position in the New York area, until on April 15, 1931, the head of the powerful Genovese family—Guiseppe Masseria, or "Joe the Boss"—was fatally wounded in a gang war. Enough was enough, and a governing body called The Commission was formed to oversee Mafia activities and settle disputes without bloodshed. This "board of directors" comprised representatives from each of the five New York families, plus two others.

In addition to the members of The Commission, there was another crime family, the DeCavalcantes, operating in New Jersey—the state where Richard Leonard Kuklinski was born on April 11, 1935. He was the second of four children,

"Assassin, it sounds so exotic. I was just a murderer." *–Richard Kuklinski*

Richard Kuklinski. *His well-groomed and neatly dressed persona is far removed from the public perception of a violent Mafia hitman.*

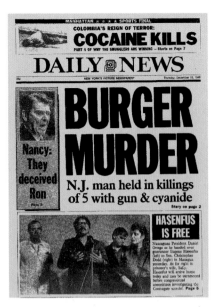

Headline news. *"Cocaine kills"* announces the Daily News—and so does a cyanide-laced burger. Kuklinski's crimes are announced to New Yorkers.

three boys and a girl. His father, Stanley, was an alcoholic Polish immigrant, prone to beating his offspring; and his mother, Anna, despite being a devout Irish Catholic, also believed in keeping her children in line, with the aid of a broom handle. The oldest child, Florian, died shortly before his eighth birthday, ostensibly after falling down a flight of stairs, but it's believed that a beating from Stanley was the real cause. This, then, was Kuklinski's world.

KUKLINSKI'S MISSPENT YOUTH

Kuklinski was only a child when he launched his homicidal career, although his early victims were feline rather than human. But as a 14-year-old he beat a neighborhood bully to death, and quickly progressed to slaughtering anyone if he didn't like the "cut of their jib"—and especially if their jib resembled his father's. Before long, the west of New York City was littered with the bodies of Kuklinski's prey, causing the police considerable perplexity. But murder was not the only outlet for Kuklinski's depravity—he threw in robbery, hijacking trucks, fencing stolen goods, and bootlegging movies for good measure.

When he was 18, Kuklinski committed a crime that would guarantee his place in the annals of Mafia history. To test his mettle, the Genovese crime family picked out a random victim and invited Kuklinski to kill him. Without hesitation, Kuklinski obliged.

KUKLINSKI TURNS PRO

Kuklinski, who was 6 feet 5 inches tall (1.95m) and heavily built, now became the Genovese family's prize hitman, although he also lent his skills to other New York families, including New Jersey's DeCavalcante family, said to have inspired the TV show *The Sopranos*. He even became the go-to assassin for "removing" senior members of the Commission to make way for new blood. When it came to murder weapons, Kuklinski was no one-trick pony—his arsenal included firearms, ice picks, hand grenades, crossbows, strangulation, even rats. When he stabbed someone, he inserted the knife into the skull, piercing the brain; this way, there was very little blood, and none at all if he left the knife in. His particular favorite, however, and the method of which he declared himself "most proud," was the nasal spray bottle filled with a cyanide solution—a quick squirt in the face and his victim was on a disoriented path to eternal rest. He'd learned the trick from another hitman, known as Mister Softee because his "day job" was selling ice cream from a van.

POISON CABINET

CYANIDE SEASONING

Kuklinski stated that he favored the cyanide method of murder because the poison is easy to administer and hard to detect. It was always wise to avoid visiting the bathroom if you were in a diner with Kuklinski, as the chances were that when you returned to the table and took a bite out of your burger, you might discover that, in your absence, he had laced it with a lethal dose of cyanide.

MODUS OPERANDI

Kuklinski was also versatile in his methods of disposing of his victims. He began by removing useful clues to identity from the body, crucially the teeth and fingers, and then tipped it into a river or a mine shaft, or broke its limbs or cut it into pieces with a chainsaw so that it would fit into a 50-gallon drum, ready to be dumped or burned (he was not fond of the chainsaw method as it left a mess, and sprayed "little pieces of meat" all over him). By way of a change, he would leave a body in a vehicle in a junkyard to be crushed by the compactor. And his pièce de résistance was placing a body in an industrial-sized freezer (another trick inspired by Mr Softee), because if the time of death cannot be established, a murderer is spared the bother of dreaming up an alibi. Kuklinski eventually came to blows with Mr Softee, and the ice-cream vendor was found dead soon afterward....

KUKLINSKI THE ROMANTIC

Kuklinski married his Italian-American girlfriend, Barbara, in 1961. He had wooed her ardently with flowers and gifts and unstinting courtesy, but when she began to feel stifled by Kuklinski and tried to back off, he stabbed her expertly—but not fatally—in the back and warned her that if she left him, he would eliminate her entire family. Needless to say, when he apologized and proposed, she agreed. It was literally an offer she couldn't refuse. She had no idea that he had already killed more than 60 men.

FAMILY GUY

Kuklinski claimed to have disliked the idea of harming women or children, but this did not inhibit him in any way when it came to beating up his wife on a regular basis. When he was in an agreeable mood, however, he was an exemplary family man, who loved Barbara and their three children, and his meerschaum pipe. He went to Mass every Sunday and served as an usher; he hosted weekly barbecues for the neighbors in the summer; he paid for his children's education, and took them on annual trips to Disneyland.

When Kuklinski was arrested as he and Barbara headed out to breakfast together, the couple had been married for 26 years. At first, Barbara had no idea why her husband was being arrested—but when a detective told her simply, "He's a murderer," she suddenly saw how everything through those 26 years added up, and knew the detective was telling the truth.

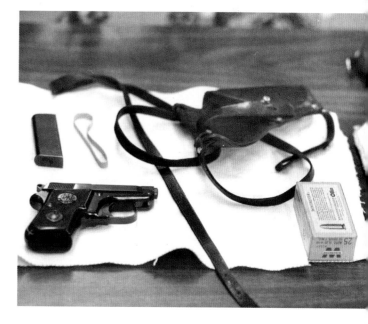

Tools of the trade. *Some of the various weapons seized by police as part of the investigation into Richard Kuklinski.*

LIFE IMPRISONMENT

The great paradox of Kuklinski was that he had his life as a contract killer and his life of suburban normality, and never the twain would meet, except for one occasion when he and Barbara socialized with a local Mafia fence, Phil Solimene, and his wife. Solimene later colluded with the task force set up to investigate Kuklinski, who had been getting careless when disposing of bodies—in particular the body that was found full of ice crystals, earning him his nickname. Kuklinski was charged with five murders. He was found guilty of four of them, and later of two more, but was never charged with the remaining 200 or so deaths for which he claimed responsibility. He spent the rest of his life in Trenton State Prison, bragging happily about his criminal exploits to anyone inclined to listen, and died on March 5, 2006. He had claimed he was being poisoned.

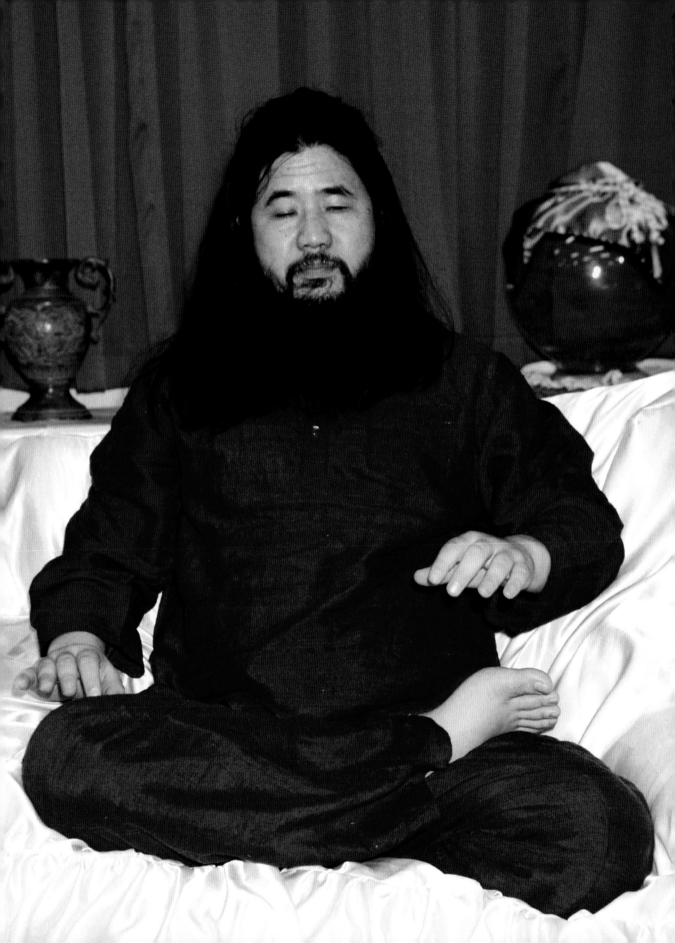

THE TOKYO SUBWAY SARIN POISONINGS

The date is March 20, 1995; the place is Tokyo, Japan. It is Monday morning rush hour, and commuters are packed into subway trains on their way to work. They do not know that they are sharing their journey with members of the doomsday cult Aum Shinrikyo, armed with plastic sacks full of the highly toxic nerve agent sarin, which they intend to release.

POISONER

Shoko Asahara
Born: March 2, 1955, Yatsushiro, Japan
Motive: Assassination, terrorism
Poison: Sarin
Number of victims: 27

SPRING IS A VERY SPECIAL TIME in Japan, and the commuters on the Tokyo subway had *sakura* to look forward to—the froth of fragrant pink cherry blossom that bursts forth in April, cheering the soul at the end of winter. But 13 of those commuters would die as a result of the attack, and many more would be blinded. They would never again take part in the joyful practice of *hanami*, strolling and picnicking beneath the trees to delight in the sight and scent of the flowers. Aum Shinrikyo had put an end to that.

AN IMPRESSIONABLE AUDIENCE

Japan is traditionally a very spiritual country, and for centuries the main religions were Shinto (based on ancestor and nature worship) and Buddhism, or a combination of the two. However, for various reasons religion took a back seat in the wake of World War II. In Russia, meanwhile, the Orthodox Church had been suppressed under Communist rule. By the end of the twentieth century, therefore, people in both countries, facing the turmoil of a rapidly changing capitalist and political landscape, were feeling in need of some theistic grounding. They were ready to embrace an inspiring new religion like Aum Shinrikyo, which promised a spiritual rebirth and even supernatural powers.

ABOUT AUM SHINRIKYO

Aum Shinrikyo was founded by Shoko Asahara, given name Chizuo Matsumoto, who was born in 1955 in Yatsushiro, Kumamoto prefecture. He was partially blind at birth and educated at a dedicated school for the blind, from which he graduated in 1975. He wanted to train as a doctor but when he failed to gain a place at medical school he compromised by studying acupuncture and pharmacology. He went on to open a pharmacy in Chiba, a city in the eponymous

Shoko Asahara. The inscrutable founder of the deadly doomsday cult Aum Shinrikyo.

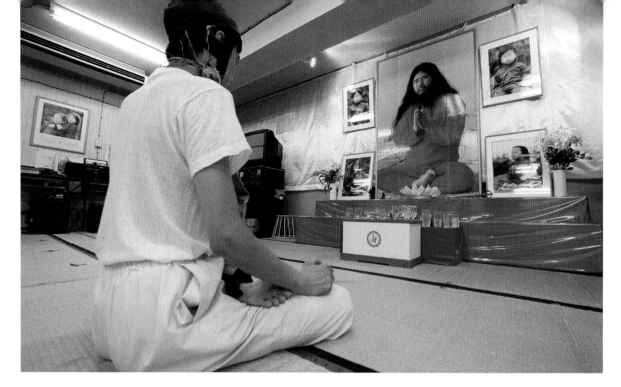

Complete devotion. *A follower of Aum Shinrikyo meditates beneath the watchful gaze of a huge image of Asahara.*

prefecture that lies adjacent to Tokyo, specializing in the remedies used in traditional Chinese medicine. He was soon to be bankrupt, however, after he was arrested in 1982 for selling fake remedies and convicted of fraud.

Meanwhile, Asahara had become a member of the new Japanese religion Agon Shu, but in 1984, after his trial, he founded his own religion, Aum Shinsen-no-Kai, later renamed Aum Shinrikyo. The name derives from the Sanskrit *aum*, which represents the universe, and *shinrikyo*, "supreme truth." Aum Shinrikyo started innocently enough as a yoga and meditation class, run by Asahara, and evolved into a spiritual group based, like Agon Shu, on a combination of Hindu and Buddhist beliefs, with elements of Christianity thrown in for good measure. Membership grew steadily, appealing to young graduates in particular who were bracing themselves for a future fraught with career pressures. However, the group started to attract controversy, with rumors of members under pressure to remain within the organization, whether they wanted to or not, and being forced to donate money. In 1989—the year the organization was granted official status as a religion—a lawyer representing families seeking to free relatives from the group was brutally murdered, along with his wife and young son.

"A series of violent phenomena filled with fear that are too difficult to describe will occur."

Shoko Asahara

AUM SHINRIKYO MOVES ON

By the early 1990s, Aum Shinrikyo had developed into a paranoid doomsday cult obsessed with Armageddon. The shift had started when Asahara began promoting himself as a reincarnation of both Jesus Christ and Gautama Buddha and as "Savior of the Country"—the country he now aspired to lead as prime minister. In 1990, he compiled a list of candidates from the Aum membership for election to the Japanese parliament, believing this to be his route to success, but the bid failed, and instead he set off along a different, far more destructive path to achieve his aim. He predicted, Nostradamus-style, that a series of disasters would occur for

Japan, including involvement in a third world war. Armageddon was imminent, he was convinced, and while he was citing the United States as the enemy who would bring about Japan's downfall, it appeared that he himself was planning to make the disasters happen, with the aim of Aum Shinrikyo replacing the government in the ensuing chaos. The organization's structure even mirrored that of the government, with ministerial departments such as the Ministry of Science and Technology.

THE PLAN OF ATTACK

Asahara's once spiritually focused group—which now had huge financial assets and an international membership running to tens of thousands, including many in Russia—began to amass AK-47 assault rifles and also acquired a Russian helicopter. Significantly, the group's chemists started to manufacture the nerve agent sarin and its even deadlier cousin, VX. In 1992, the organization sent a 40-strong medical group to Zaire (now the Democratic Republic of the Congo), supposedly to assist in the aid program during an outbreak of Ebola but actually to attempt to obtain the virus to add to Aum's growing arsenal of biochemical weapons. Fortunately, their quest failed.

In June 1994, the group released sarin gas from a specially adapted vehicle parked near a dormitory where judges presiding over a case against Aum were staying, along with other court officials. The judges survived the attack, although they were injured along with many others, but eight people died. The authorities suspected Aum but were unable to take any action as the organization was protected by its religious status. The magnitude of the next attack would well and truly overshadow this one, and there were more in the pipeline—including, it later emerged, a plan to spray sarin over the city from that Russian helicopter.

THE TOKYO SUBWAY ATTACK

The execution of the Tokyo subway attack was stunning in its simplicity. On the morning of March 20, 1995, five Aum members—all graduates or holding postgraduate degrees—boarded separate subway trains on three different lines heading for Kasumigaseki station, carefully synchronizing the timing of their journeys to ride trains that would converge there simultaneously. The station lies in the heart of Japan's national administration and politics district, a short distance from the National Diet Building on Kasumigaseki Hill (home of the Japanese parliament), various government agencies, and the Imperial Palace, so the passengers on the train were a perfect fit for the terrorists' target profile.

POISON CABINET

Sarin, a colorless, odorless, and extremely toxic liquid, has only been used a few times in history. Exposure to it is lethal in minutes even at very low concentrations.

It was first developed in Nazi Germany in the 1930s by scientists in search of a more potent pesticide, but despite its efficacy, it was not used as a weapon against the Allies in World War II. Asahara's role model was none other than Hitler himself, and he too visualized a world peopled only by himself and his followers.

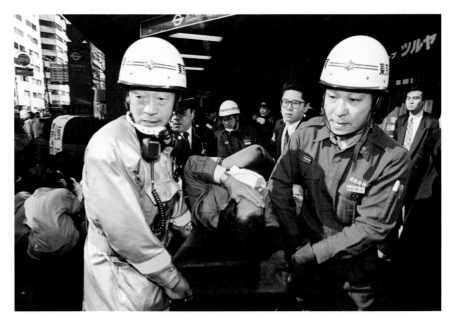

Subway attack. *Members of the rescue team hurry a blinded victim away for treatment after the gas attack.*

The terrorists each carried a plastic sack containing a quantity of liquid sarin, disguised beneath a loosely folded newspaper, and an umbrella with a sharp metal tip. At prearranged stations near Kasumigaseki, all the terrorists placed their newspapers on the floor and pierced the plastic sacks several times with the tips of their umbrellas. Then they simply left their respective stations and were whisked away in waiting cars, leaving the colorless, odorless toxin to seep from the sacks, permeate the trains, and do its deadly work.

THE AFTERMATH

The devastation the terrorists left behind was horrific, worthy of an Oscar-winning movie—except that this was real. Commuters affected by the toxin staggered from the trains and fell onto the platforms, dizzy, blinded, gasping for breath, some with blood flooding from their noses and mouths, all desperate to reach the exits and escape to the open air above ground. And soon they were joined by members of the chemical warfare unit, clad from head to toe in protective gear, whose job was to neutralize the poison, which was not well understood at the time.

A total of 13 people died as a direct result of the attack, and more than 6,000 others suffered the effects of the sarin. Many made a full recovery, but many others were left with permanent damage to their eyes, lungs, and digestive systems, and nearly a third of those who were traveling on the trains to Kasumigaseki were still suffering from post-traumatic stress disorder 20 years later, reporting feeling insecure whenever they had to ride a train. The only consolation is that it could have been so much worse had the sarin been deployed by a different method, with the death toll potentially running to thousands.

RENEWAL

In the year 2000, around 1,500 members of Aum Shinrikyo reformed, naming themselves Aleph (the first letter of the Hebrew and Arabic alphabet, signifying "renewal") under the leadership of Jōyū Fumihiro. Aleph continued to operate as a spiritual group, apologizing to the victims of the Tokyo subway bombing and setting up a compensation fund. In 2007, Jōyū Fumihiro left Aleph and formed a splinter organization—Hikari no Wa, meaning "Circle of Light"—with around 150 members. Both groups were placed under government surveillance because of their direct association with the original Aum Shinrikyo cult.

THE MANHUNT

It was not long before suspicion fell on Aum Shinrikyo, and the ensuing hunt for the terrorists proved to be one of the largest in Japan's history. Within days of the attack, squads of helmeted riot police began raids on known Aum facilities around the country, and there they discovered all the ingredients for extensive chemical and biological attacks. They had found their culprits. Hundreds of cult members were arrested immediately. Asahara proved more elusive, but was tracked down on May 16 at the cult's headquarters, meditating alone in a secret room. His arrest, which he accepted without protest, was broadcast live. Eventually, around 200 cult members were convicted in connection with the Tokyo subway attack and earlier incidents. The last to be tried was not tracked down until 2012, after 17 years on the run. He was sentenced to life imprisonment.

Aum was quickly stripped of its official status as a "religious legal entity," although it was not actually banned, and within two years the authorities had done such an effective job of undermining its financial base and discrediting its ideology that its days as a terrorist organization were, apparently, over. However, although it was outlawed in its other main base, Russia, the cult still survives there, according to reports published in 2016, and is causing concern; and in other countries, including the USA, Aum is a designated terrorist organization.

THE VERDICT

On February 27, 2004, Asahara was sentenced to death by hanging for the murder of 27 people in thirteen separate indictments. Twelve other cult members were also sentenced to death and others received life imprisonment. In 2016, the Supreme Court dismissed a final appeal on behalf of Asahara, affirming that he is legally sane and thus can be held responsible for his actions, although his defense team protested the ruling, insisting that the psychological examination that found him to be mentally competent was "flawed." To date, Asahara remains in solitary confinement, awaiting the execution date to be set. He might have fallen far short of his goal, but he certainly made his mark, in the worst of all possible ways.

Wanted poster. *Police search for three people believed to be involved in the biological attack—a daily reminder to Tokyo commuters.*

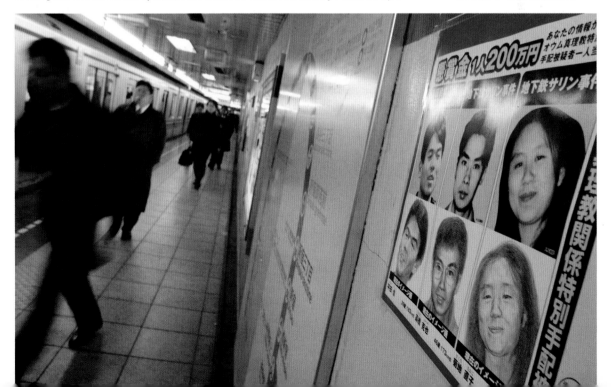

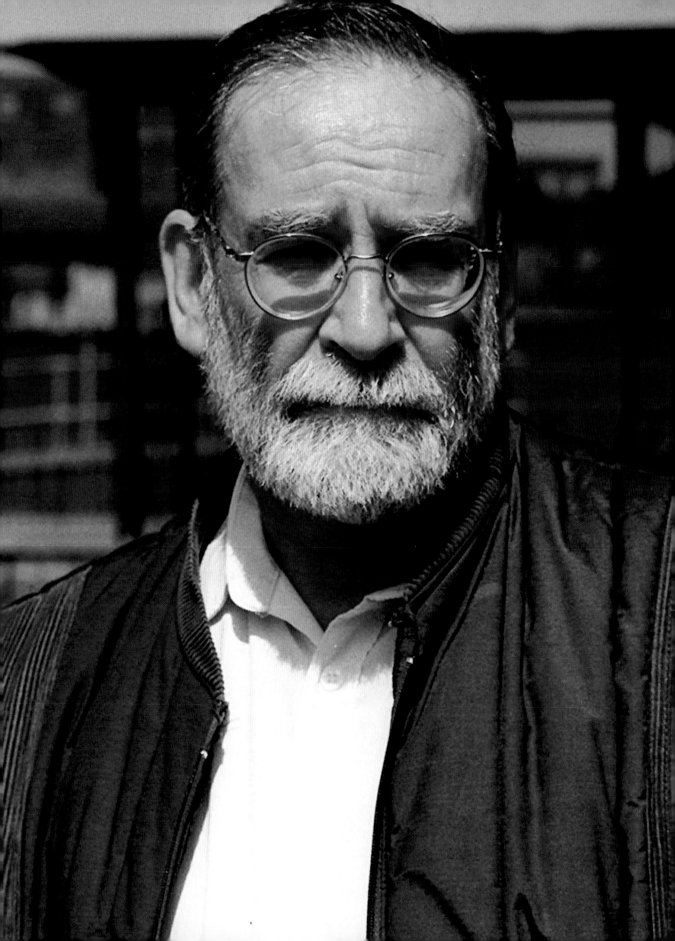

HAROLD SHIPMAN
Dr Death Comes Calling

It's the worst nightmare imaginable: a doctor, entrusted with his patients' health and under oath to do no harm, goes rogue. The case of Dr Harold Shipman, the most prolific serial killer in British history, is a very dark one indeed. Yet his crimes went undetected for over two decades and—perhaps most shocking of all—they were finally uncovered by accident.

POISONER

Harold Frederick Shipman
Born: January 14, 1946, Nottingham, England
Died: January 13, 2004, by suicide in Wakefield Prison, Yorkshire, England
Motive: Unknown
Poison: Morphine
Number of victims: At least 215, possibly up to 260

TRACKING A FORGERY

ON JUNE 24, 1998, Kathleen Grundy died at her home in Hyde, on the outskirts of Manchester, England. She had been a lively, sociable woman, a previous mayoress of Hyde and a tireless worker for elderly people, and, although she was 81 years old, she had seemed to be in robust health. It was therefore rather unexpected when she was found dead, sitting in a chair, a cold cup of tea at her side, but her doctor, Harold Shipman, confirmed that that she had died from heart failure.

Kathleen's daughter Angela accepted the explanation—after all, her mother had been elderly. But a week or two later she was surprised to be contacted by a firm of local lawyers with a copy of what they claimed was Kathleen's will. Angela, a lawyer herself, was close to her mother and had always managed her legal affairs. The will was clumsily typed and the signature did not look like Kathleen's—and it left all her mother's money to Harold Shipman. Angela, who had previously drawn up a will for her mother, believed it was fraudulent and called the police. It did not take long to trace the will back to the doctor, its sole proposed beneficiary—the machine it had been typed on was found in a cupboard at his office.

The forged will prompted questions about Kathleen's death. Shipman had advised her family that no autopsy was needed, so they had gone ahead with arrangements for her funeral, which had already taken place. With suspicions of foul play growing, orders were given for Kathleen's body to be exhumed on August 1. It was found to contain enough morphine to have killed her. Police called Shipman in for questioning and on September 7 he was charged both with the murder of Mrs Grundy and the forging of her will. The process of unmasking the caring family doctor was just beginning and the revelations to come of Shipman's crimes would shock the community, and the wider world.

Dr Harold Shipman. *The doctor's calm, rather scholarly façade masked the worst serial killer in British history.*

THE MAKING OF A MURDERER

Where had Dr Shipman come from?

Harold Frederick Shipman, "Fred" to his friends and colleagues, had apparently had a rather ordinary start in life. His father was a truck driver, but his aspirational son worked hard to get into the prestigious local school where he was known as a quiet, calm boy who was also an enthusiastic athlete and rugby player.

He was studying for his college exams when his mother, who had suffered from lung cancer for some years, died. Outwardly her death did not seem to affect his plans for the future; he managed to gain a place at medical school in Leeds, Yorkshire, from where he graduated after five years, along the way marrying his 17-year-old girlfriend, Primrose Oxtoby. The couple would go on to have four children; friends noticed that Shipman was very much master of his household, with the shy, quiet Primrose tending to defer to his opinions.

By the early 1970s, Shipman's medical career seemed to be well on track. After a stint as a junior hospital doctor, he joined a general practice in Todmorden, West Yorkshire. In a group of mostly older doctors, he was seen as modern and forward thinking; one patient recalled, years later, that he was rather glamorous. "It was just so cool having a young attractive doctor there," she said "(He) looked like the doctors on television." After several apparently uneventful years, however, the practice found that quantities of pethidine, a powerful painkiller, were going missing from the surgery, and the culprit was eventually found to be Shipman. Cornered, he confessed to having formed an addiction and went into rehab.

> "Never at the beginning of that investigation did I envisage that I would be dealing with not only one murder investigation but a number of murder investigations."
>
> *Detective Stan Egerton*

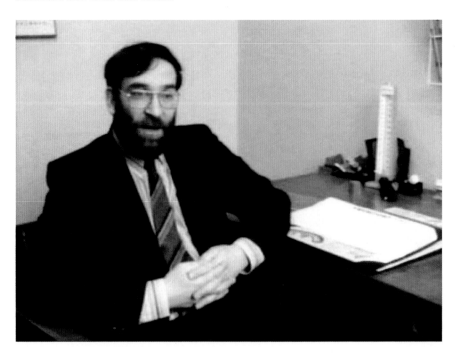

Family doctor. *Pictured in his surgery in the 1980s, Shipman was known in Hyde as a popular, hardworking GP. At one point, he was even interviewed for the British television program* World in Action *about the benefits of a "care in the community" policy.*

The setback did not seem to harm his career. Completing rehab less than a year after his addiction had been uncovered, he moved to Hyde with Primrose and their family, joining the Donneybrook practice there in 1977. Still only 31 years old, he was open about his previous addiction and was admired by his new colleagues for facing up to and dealing with his problems. He remained with this group practice until 1992, when he set up his own surgery in the town as a solo practitioner.

"NOTHING WAS TOO MUCH TROUBLE"

Dr Shipman proved particularly popular with older patients. While other busy doctors always seemed short of time and were keen on encouraging people to come to the surgery wherever possible, he had more old-fashioned habits. The elderly noted approvingly that he was never too busy to pay them a visit at home; younger people admired his patience with their older family members. Locally, he had a big fan club—everyone agreed that he really took the trouble to set his patients' minds at ease as well as to treat their ailments.

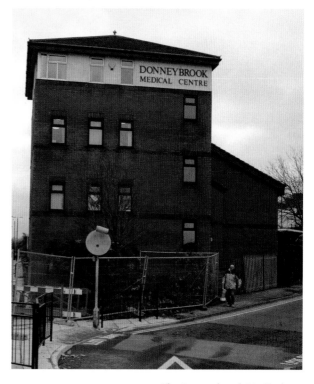

The Donneybrook Medical Centre. *It was while he was working at this practice that attention was first drawn to the very high number of deaths among Shipman's patients.*

But in 1988, nearly a decade after Shipman came to Hyde, a local funeral director, Deborah Massey, noticed that there was a remarkably high mortality rate among his patients. Not only that, but there were some troubling similarities about the manner of their deaths. Most were older women who had been found at home, dressed, and sitting on a chair. They were not ill in bed; their deaths tended to be unexpected. Shipman completed death certificates giving heart failure, or in some cases simply old age, as the cause. The coroner had a discreet look at Shipman's practice but eventually concluded that the high death rate was because he had more elderly patients on his list than most other doctors. It had been a chance to catch Shipman—but it was missed. He would not be stopped for another ten years.

Other people were to notice the high death rate among Shipman's patients, but they never seemed to put two and two together. His reputation as a caring,

HOW MANY DID HE KILL?
The true total of Shipman's victims will probably never be known. An official inquiry in 2002—carried out by making a clinical audit into over 800 deaths, some dating from his days in practice at Todmorden—concluded that in his 24 years in practice as a doctor he had killed "at least" 215 people, with the possibility that the total might actually be closer to 260. Other researchers put the totals at 300, or even more. Nor can we know when he started killing—he may even have begun as a young hospital houseman. Even at 215 victims, he has the dubious distinction of being not only Britain's worst serial killer—by far—but also a contender for the worst confirmed serial killer anywhere in the world.

conscientious practitioner was widely known and respected. As he moved into his 40s, he cultivated the look of a genial, relaxed authority figure, with tweed jackets, a bushy beard, and thick glasses. His readiness to pay house calls added to his popularity. And his older patients kept on dying.

Four months before Kathleen Grundy's death, another local doctor had prompted the start of a secret police inquiry into Harold Shipman. In England, if a body is to be cremated, two doctors need to sign the certificate— and she had noticed how many certificates she was signing on which Dr Shipman was the first signatory. The police started a very discreet investigation, but it had not progressed far at the point at which the investigation into Kathleen Grundy's death began. She was to be Shipman's final victim.

THE KILLER UNMASKED

Police questioning Shipman found him uncooperative. At first, he replied with an incredulous "How dare you?" When that failed to convince, he behaved as though the detectives were somehow unqualified to question him; the senior detective who first arrested and later charged Shipman, Stan Egerton, remembered the doctor as arrogant and tetchy, conveying the impression that he would have expected to be questioned by a detective inspector at the very least. Shipman admitted nothing, but searches of his home and surgery quickly uncovered collections of random items from his supposed victims, mostly small pieces of jewelry and keepsakes, and his computer records relating to suspicious deaths had been backdated and falsified. When the evidence of the records was put to Shipman, he collapsed and his solicitor had further interviews suspended for some weeks. On his return, he responded to most inquiries with "no comment." He never again answered a direct police question.

"None of your victims realized that yours was not a healing touch."

Judge John Forbes

Meanwhile, the horror was mounting. There was soon enough evidence to order further exhumations, and eventually 12 bodies were exhumed. It was clear that Harold Shipman's crimes went far, far beyond anything that had previously been suspected. More and more evidence established that he had a "typical" method. He would attend one of his patients, usually an older person who lived alone, at home, either by prior appointment, for some relatively minor complaint, or without an appointment, unexpectedly. In the course of the visit and under some pretext of a treatment that they needed the doctor would inject them with a dose of morphine sufficient to kill them. He would then usually leave, either returning to "discover" the body later, or allowing others to do so. He killed men and women, although more than two-thirds of his victims were women, most over the age of 60, and many much older. He ascribed many deaths to heart failure, although with his oldest victims he would sometimes simply write "old age" on the death certificate. He did this repeatedly, often without arousing any suspicion whatsoever. He killed his victims in their own homes and in care homes; he is even believed to have killed five patients in the course of their visits to his surgery. In one particularly chilling instance he recorded a patient's death before going out to kill her.

KATHLEEN GRUNDY
LOUGHRIGG COTTAGE
79 JOEL LANE
HYDE
CHESHIRE
SKI4 5JZ

RECEIVED 2 4 JUN 1998

22.6.98

Dear Sir,

I enclose a copy of my will. I think it is clear in intent. I wish Dr. shipman to benefit by having my estate but if he dies or cannot accept it ,then the estate goes to my daughter.
I would like you to be the executor of the will, I intend to make an appointment to discuss this and my will in the near future.
Yours sincerely

K. Grundy.

A step too far. *The purported will of Kathleen Grundy. Clumsily typed, it was easily identified as a forgery, but was it a sign that Harold Shipman really wanted to be stopped?*

Why did he do it? None of the labels used for Shipman—and he was to be variously defined as a psychopath, a sociopath, and a narcissist—go any way toward offering a real reason. Despite the small thefts, money was evidently not a motive; as for the clumsy will forgery, most criminal psychologists seemed to see it as a subconscious attempt to be caught and stopped. Criminologists gave lengthy interviews about him. Some suggested that teenage memories of seeing his mother being injected with morphine as she lay dying had had long-term traumatic effects. But Shipman kept his lip firmly buttoned. For a man so arrogant, it is possible that simply proving his power to choose life or death for his patients was enough to trigger his killer impulses.

TRIAL AND CONVICTION

Harold Shipman went on trial at Preston Crown Court on October 5, 1999, charged with forgery and 15 counts of murder. He put in a not guilty plea, but was convicted on all charges on January 31, 2000. It was decided not to charge him with any of the other murders he had undoubtedly committed, because, given the immense public interest in the case, it would be impossible to give him a fair trial. He was sentenced to "full-term life," meaning that there was no possibility that he would ever leave prison.

The verdict left the public reeling. How was it possible that a doctor could have killed such a huge number of people? Why had more warning signs not been spotted, nor seriously pursued? Long opinion pieces appeared in the newspapers discussing the role of older people in society and questioning whether it was the age of his victims that had seemed to make them so invisible.

Dr Shipman kept his counsel and continued to refuse interviews. In jail he became known for offering medical advice to elderly fellow prisoners, although it is hard to imagine that anyone would have taken it. Early on the morning of January 13, 2004, the day before his 58th birthday, he made a noose from his bedsheets and hanged himself from the bars of his cell in Wakefield Prison in Yorkshire. It had always been important to him to stay in control, and he remained in control—as far as possible—to the bitter end.

Front page news. *Shipman's trial and its shocking conclusions dominated both the local and national news in the UK for weeks.*

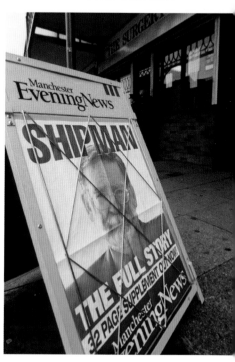

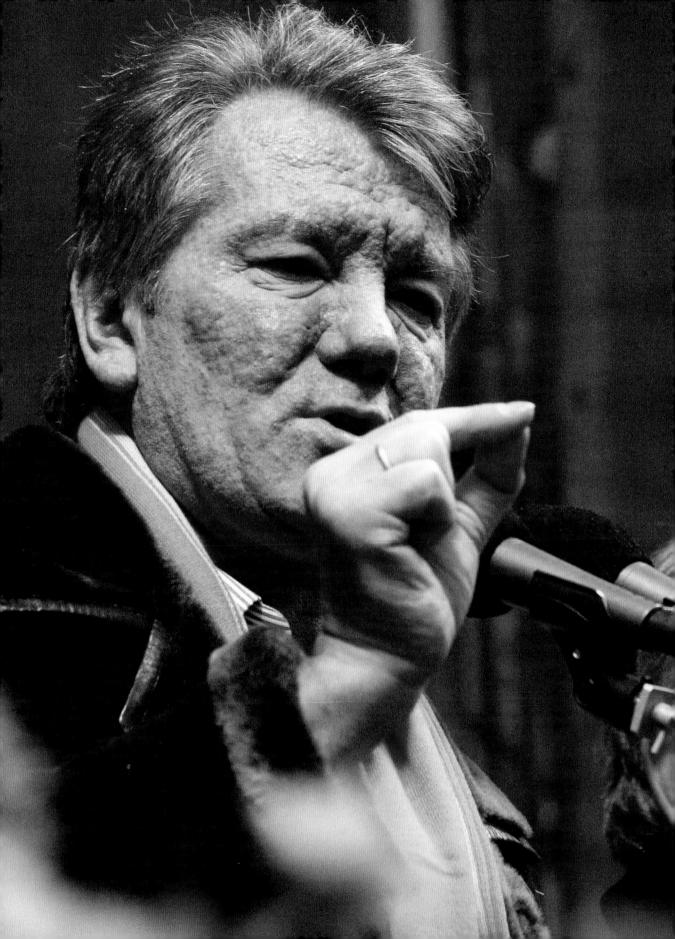

VIKTOR YUSHCHENKO
Dioxin Disfigurement

No one expects to eat a bowl of soup and end up with a face disfigured by a blotchy mask of lesions and blisters, but that is exactly what happened to the handsome Ukrainian opposition leader Viktor Yushchenko shortly before the 2004 presidential elections. So what exactly was in that soup—and was it meant to kill him?

VIKTOR YUSHCHENKO was born on February 23, 1954, in the village of Khoruzhivka in the Sumy region of northern Ukraine. In 1975, he graduated with a degree in economic sciences from the Ternopil Finance and Economics Faculty of the Kyiv [Kiev] National Economic University, and this would set him on a career path in the field of banking—and ultimately politics—at a very significant moment in Ukraine's history.

A SPIRITED PEOPLE

The area known today as Ukraine has a history dating back thousands of years, and by the eleventh century CE the powerful state of Kievan Rus, with the prosperous city of Kiev at its heart, was geographically the largest in Europe. However, warring factions divided the state, and in 1240 Kiev was besieged by marauding Mongols continuing the campaign of plunder, conquest, and empire-building begun by their infamous late warrior-ruler, Genghis Khan; the old city was razed and almost the entire population was massacred. During the following century, the territory was annexed by Poland and Lithuania, but far from breaking the spirit of the Ukrainian people, this made them stronger and more culturally united, an attitude that sustained them through a prolonged period of partitioning. This concluded in 1793, when most of Ukraine was integrated into the rapidly expanding Russian Empire, while the extreme west of the region fell under the control of the Austro-Hungarian Empire.

Still the Ukrainian spirit refused to be subjugated, and in the early nineteenth century the people resolved to revive their linguistic and cultural traditions, and even to reestablish a Ukrainian state—an ambition that was firmly quashed by Imperial Russia. Revolution was brewing, however, and the Russian Empire fell in 1917. Meanwhile, the Austro-Hungarian Empire had also been disintegrating during World War I, and was dissolved in 1918. Ukraine seized its chance, reunited

Viktor Yushchenko. *Pockmarked but proud, Yushchenko pictured in orange, his campaign color.*

its two territories, and declared independent statehood—but again it was to prove nothing more than an ambition, as Ukraine was officially incorporated into the Soviet Union in 1922.

There followed more than half a century of extremely difficult times, during which Ukraine endured traumas such as forced collectivization under Stalin, Nazi occupation during World War II, and the 1986 nuclear disaster at the Chernobyl Power Plant, which caused the deaths of tens of thousands of people, along with major economic and ecological damage. By now, however, the Soviet Union was starting to crumble, and the phoenix that was Ukrainian nationalism began to rise once more, albeit cautiously, from the ashes. Russification was out; Ukrainian culture was in. On July 16, 1990, the Declaration of State Sovereignty of Ukraine was passed, followed on August 24, 1991, by the Declaration of Independence. In December of that year, the Ukrainian people voted overwhelmingly for full independence in a referendum and Leonid Kravchuk became the first democratically elected president of Ukraine. In July 1994 he lost reelection to Leonid Kuchma, who would shape Yushchenko's future in politics.

> "What happened to me was an attempt to politically destroy a politician with opposing views." —*Viktor Yushchenko*

YUSHCHENKO'S METEORIC RISE

After graduation, Yushchenko returned to Sumy, where his first job was as an accounting assistant on a *kolkhoz*, one of the collective farms that had caused so much grief to the Ukrainian peasantry when collectivization—the compulsory relinquishing of individual farms to form large units—was established between 1929 and 1933. The following year, after a brief stint in the Soviet army, Yushchenko took up a position as an economist in the local branch of the Soviet State Bank. But he was destined for greater things—by the late 1980s, when the great resurgence of Ukrainian nationalism was under way, he was serving as deputy chairman of the board of directors of the Agro-Industrial Bank of Ukraine. From 1990 to 1993, the period of transition to independence,

Proud to be independent. *The Ukraine Pro-Independence rally held in 1991, the year the country's 70-year membership of the Soviet Union came to an end.*

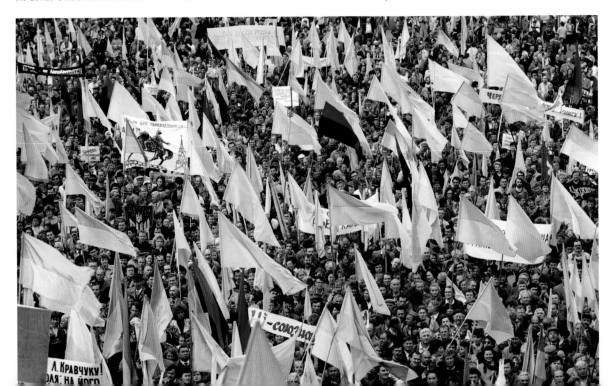

Yushchenko was the first deputy chairman of the board of Bank Ukraina, then in 1993, at the age of 39, he was appointed governor of the National Bank of Ukraine. Here he would oversee the introduction in 1996 of the national currency, the *hryvnia*, a modern transliteration of *grivna*, the currency (and measure of weight) of medieval Kievan Rus. It was all part of the cultural revival.

YUSHCHENKO TAKES TO POLITICS

In 1999, Yushchenko was appointed prime minister by Leonid Kuchma, the second president of independent Ukraine. Kuchma, a former engineer, was in his second term as president, although his failure to improve the country's economy had made him less than popular and there had been claims of voting irregularities in the 1999 election. Yushchenko, with his background in banking, was a clever choice—he was an advocate of economic reform, and within 18 months had brought in strict measures such as ending the practice of providing subsidies to unprofitable companies. Indeed, for Kuchma he was proving too clever a choice, credited as he was with helping Ukraine to emerge from its economic doldrums where Kuchma had failed, and in 2001 he was summarily dismissed as prime minister.

OUR UKRAINE

Dismissing Yushchenko served only to spur him into action, and his response was to form a democratic coalition party called "Our Ukraine." The party took the biggest share of the vote in the parliamentary elections held in March 2002, reflecting support for democratic reforms, but despite this the elections ended in the formation of a government principally loyal to Kuchma. Within a year, however, opinion polls indicated that an overwhelming majority of Ukrainians had had their fill of Kuchma, who was being held responsible for the country's economic ruin. He was also accused of using intimidation to undermine his opponents and force them to surrender their allegiance to democratic parties. But among his opponents was a very determined Viktor Yushchenko, whose next goal was victory in the presidential elections to be held in 2004.

UKRAINE'S POLITICAL CUISINE

Fast-forward to September 5, 2004, and we find Yushchenko in Kiev, meeting over dinner with the chairman and deputy chairman of the Ukrainian Security Service (SBU) to discuss the role of the security services in the election campaign. By the following day, Yushchenko was experiencing stomach pains; he was examined by Ukrainian doctors and declared to be suffering from food poisoning. When he had failed to show any sign of recovery by September 10, he was taken to the Rudolfinerhaus, a private clinic in Vienna with an outstanding international reputation for both medicine and technical innovation. Yushchenko

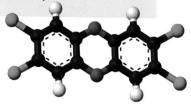

Dioxin. *A diagram showing the complex chemical structure of* TCDD, *which was classified in 1997 as a carcinogen in humans.*

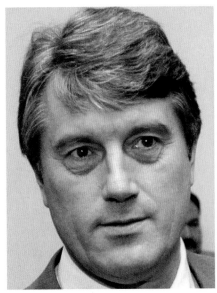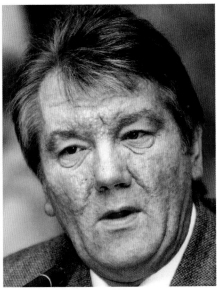

Before and after. *The damage wrought on the politician's handsome face by a dose of dioxin.*

was examined by no fewer than 11 doctors, who diagnosed acute pancreatitis accompanied by interstitial edematous changes—which translated into layman's terms meant that his liver, pancreas, and intestines were swollen and his digestive tract was severely ulcerated.

With the presidential election imminent, this could not have happened at a worse time, and—ignoring the advice of the medics—Yushchenko returned to the campaign trail. By now he suspected that an attempt had been made on his life, and on September 21 he declared that he had fallen victim to "Ukraine's political cuisine which kills." His main rival, Kuchma's prime minister, Viktor Yanukovych, asserted that he "knew nothing," accusing Yushchenko in return of gorging himself on bad sushi and an excess of alcohol.

THE DISFIGUREMENT OF YUSHCHENKO

On September 30, Yushchenko returned to Vienna, complaining of severe back pain. When next he hit the campaign trail, he was receiving painkillers directly into his spine via a catheter. But this was to prove the least of Yushchenko's problems. Two weeks after the dinner, he had begun to suffer from severe facial edema. Three weeks later, his face was still puffy, paralyzed on the left side, and now small nodular lesions had appeared, which rapidly developed into painful, inflamed cysts, giving Yushchenko the appearance of someone suffering from a bad attack of acne. Lesions then started to appear on his body, and by nine months after the dinner they had spread to his entire body.

THE DIOXIN DEBATE

Uncomfortable and unsightly they may have been, but those lesions provided the vital clue to solving the mystery. Images of Yushchenko's almost unrecognizable face appeared around the world, prompting a debate among the

SAVING FACE

In 2009, *New Scientist* magazine reported that, in the opinion of doctors at the Swiss Centre for Human Applied Toxicology, who had been treating and monitoring Yushchenko since the incident five years earlier, those disfiguring skin growths had possibly saved the politician's life by isolating the dioxin from vital internal organs. The skin is already a major organ of detoxification, but the growths, called "hamartomas," were effectively a new organ, created from the existing skin stem cells, that expressed very high levels of dioxin-metabolizing enzymes.

medical community as to the cause. A toxicologist at a London hospital identified the marks on Yushchenko's face as chloracne, and suggested they were the result of dioxin poisoning. A clinical scientist at another London hospital concurred that chloracne is a side effect of dioxin, but argued that he had never heard of dioxin being used as a "malicious chemical agent." Meanwhile, an American professor of dermatology proposed rosacea, which can be triggered by stress and often leaves the face looking swollen and lumpy.

But it was the toxicologist who was proved to be right. Doctors at the clinic in Vienna consulted experts in the USA, and on December 11 announced that Yushchenko had indeed been poisoned with dioxin, possibly administered in the soup served at the dinner in Kiev. A minute amount secreted in food is enough to cause severe illness and had the dose been any higher, Yushchenko might well have died—and had he died before the lesions appeared, the truth might never have been revealed. In the event, his long-term prognosis was pronounced to be good—so perhaps this was not so much a genuine assassination attempt as a warning shot.

> "If someone put a drop of pure dioxin in his food, he wouldn't taste it, he wouldn't see it…"
>
> *Arnold Schecter, dioxin expert*

THE ORANGE REVOLUTION

Meanwhile, the first round of the presidential election had been held on October 31. Neither Viktor emerged the victor, with Yushchenko and Yanukovych each winning around 40 percent of the vote, necessitating a runoff. This was held on November 21 and Yanukovych was declared the winner, sparking a cry of "fraud" by Yushchenko's supporters and nearly two weeks of mass protests that came to be known as the Orange Revolution—not a reflection of the Agent Orange connection, but because orange was Yushchenko's campaign color.

The Supreme Court overturned the result on the grounds of poll fraud, and another runoff was held on December 26. This time, Yushchenko received a winning 52 percent of the vote, and was inaugurated on January 23, 2005—pockmarked, but proud.

The Orange Revolution.
The vociferous mass protests of 2004 contributed to a successful result for Yushchenko.

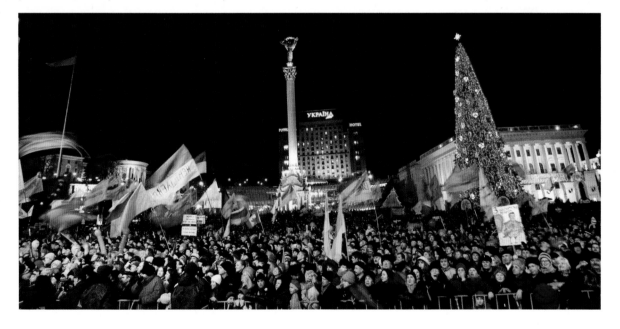

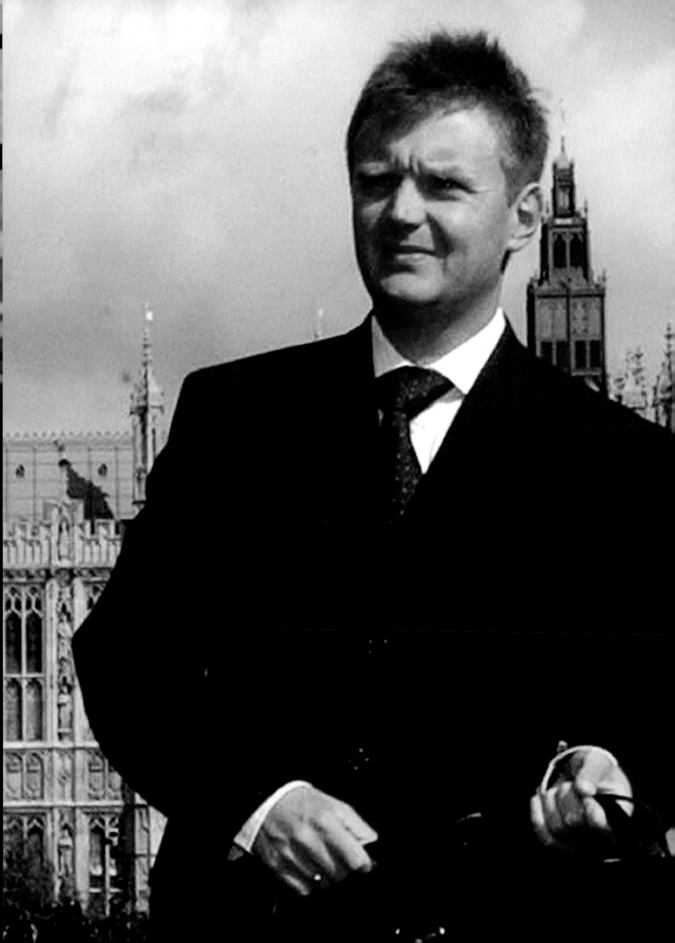

ALEXANDER LITVINENKO
Assassinated in London

On November 17, 2006, Scotland Yard officers were summoned to the bedside of a patient in intensive care at University College Hospital in London. They were given very little idea of what to expect. The man had been transferred from the general hospital near his home in north London. On admission, he had given his name as Edwin Carter and he appeared to be suffering from some form of acute poisoning. Nothing could have prepared the doctors for the extraordinary story that he had to tell.

THE PATIENT SPOKE reasonably good English, but it was heavily accented and unidiomatic—it clearly was not his mother tongue. And it soon became clear why—his real name was not Edwin Carter, but Alexander Litvinenko. He had been a Russian security agent. And as would later be made clear at the public enquiry into his death held in London in 2016, he believed he had been poisoned on Russian orders.

THE PATH TO POISON

At the time of the poisoning, Alexander Litvinenko had recently become a British citizen. He had been born in Voronezh, about 300 miles (483 kilometers) south of Moscow, and had served in the Russian army before being transferred to the KGB, the Russian security services, in 1988. He worked for the KGB—renamed the FSB in 1994—until 1999. After spending some time in their anti-terrorist unit, he was moved to a job investigating organized crime within Russia, a role that would make him many enemies and one he took to with enthusiasm. Corruption was rife in Russia but he was fearless in calling people to account, and he was highly critical of many of the Kremlin's policies. Vladimir Putin was head of the FSB while Litvinenko worked there, and the two reportedly clashed during that time.

In 1998, Litvinenko's FSB career came to an end when, at a press conference he openly accused the FSB of ordering him to murder Boris Berezovsky, an oligarch and businessman who had been close to President Boris Yeltsin and was a vocal critic of Putin. It led to his arrest and imprisonment for a year, and shortly after his release, Litvinenko fled to Britain with his family, claiming political

Alexander Litvinenko. *In exile, but healthy and confident, he had fingers in many business and surveillance pies.*

asylum. Once in London he kept his fingers in a wide variety of pies, working in different capacities, including as a writer, a journalist and a "consultant" for various parties. Boris Berezovsky, also in exile in England, gave him financial support, helping with the school fees of his son, Anatoly. Less publically, Litvinenko was reportedly paid a retainer by MI6. It is believed that he gave them information on the links between senior Kremlin officials and organized crime in Russia. Even in London, the life he was living was far from risk-free. He was a constant thorn in the side of the Russian administration, and he had access to enough hard information to make his widely published criticisms of Putin, now president of Russia, convincing. In the fall of 2006, he is also believed to have been investigating organized Russian crime in Spain.

"Later on, when I left the hotel, I was thinking there was something strange."

Alexander Litvinenko, giving his statement to police

A POISONING IN PUBLIC

Early on the afternoon of November 1, Litvinenko arrived for a meeting at the offices of an intelligence firm in London's exclusive Mayfair district. He had a meeting there with a man called Andrei Lugovoi, whom he had known in Moscow back in the 1990s, when both men had worked for Berezovsky. They had met again in 2005, when Lugovoi had suggested joining forces to give advice to firms who wished to invest in Russia; they could supply due diligence reports and Litvinenko could earn some extra money. Also at the meeting was an associate of Lugovoi, named Dmitri Kovtun.

It was a short meeting during which it seems Litvinenko did not drink the tea that he was served. After about half an hour, Litvinenko, Lugovoi, and Kovtun left together and moved on to a sushi bar that Litvinenko often visited in Piccadilly, where he was due to meet another associate, a man named Mario Scaramella, a rather shadowy figure who was allegedly an Italian security consultant, for whom Litvinenko was supposedly obtaining information about possible Russian influence in the recent Italian elections.

Dying in University College Hospital. *Litvinenko asked that he be photographed and the photographs published: shocking evidence of what had happened to him.*

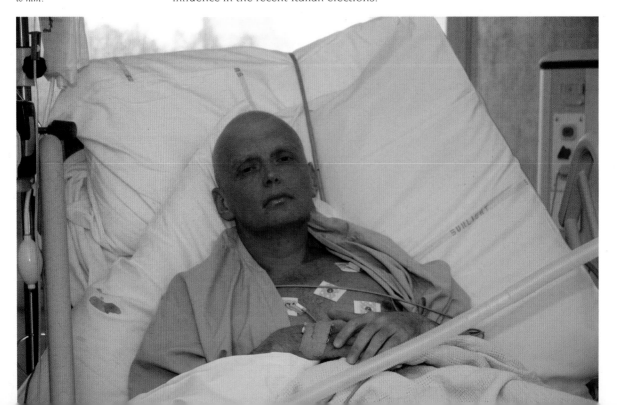

Lugovoi and Kovtun left Litvinenko with Scaramella, but not before they had arranged to meet up again later in the afternoon, apparently to discuss business. So at 4pm Litvinenko went to meet the two Russians at the Millennium Hotel in upmarket Mayfair.

The meeting took place in the Pine Bar off the hotel's foyer, almost the only public space in the hotel without CCTV, so the police were reliant on Litvinenko's direct account of what had happened there. He told them that when he arrived, he had joined Lugovoi and Kovtun in the bar. They ordered drinks; Litvinenko did not drink alcohol and was also on a tight budget—he didn't want to order in such an expensive hotel. A pot of green tea with honey and lemon was served but Litvinenko took only a few sips. He didn't finish his cup. "Maybe in total I swallowed three or four times," he would tell detectives, "I didn't like it for some reason ... well, almost cold tea with no sugar."

In addition to attending business meetings, Lugovoi was also in London to attend a soccer match—CSKA Moscow were playing Arsenal on November 2, and he'd brought his whole family—his wife, both his daughters, and his son, to see them. And at the end of the meeting he made a point of introducing his 8-year-old son to Litvinenko.

But when the latter left the hotel after less than half an hour, having made an appointment to meet up with Lugovoi yet again the following day, Litvinenko was already dying. He didn't know it yet, but a single mouthful of the tea would have been more than enough to kill him. Much later, it would be found to have contained polonium, a poison which, when ingested, has a lethal dose of less than a millionth of a gram.

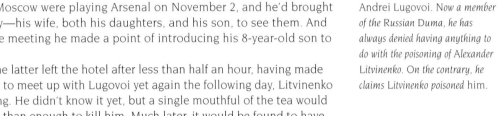

Andrei Lugovoi. *Now a member of the Russian Duma, he has always denied having anything to do with the poisoning of Alexander Litvinenko. On the contrary, he claims Litvinenko poisoned* him.

A SLOW DEATH

Alexander Litvinenko went home. Over the next two days he had a case of what looked like very bad food poisoning, with constant vomiting and diarrhea. Three days later and still no better, he was admitted to his local hospital and, when he

WHAT HAPPENED NEXT?
Andrei Lugovoi had returned to Moscow two days after the meetings with Litvinenko. Both he and Dmitri Kovtun, who is now a businessman in Moscow, have flatly denied being involved in the poisoning of Alexander Litvinenko and accused the British government and the board of the inquiry into Litvinenko's death of being complicit in a cover-up. On hearing Lugovoi described as an "ex-KGB agent," however, a colleague laughed. "There is no such thing as an ex-KGB agent," he said. Both Kovtun and Lugovoi were treated for radiation poisoning in Moscow; both turned the tables in accusing Litvinenko, possibly in association with MI6, of having poisoned them.

POISON CABINET

POLONIUM

Element 84 in the periodic table, polonium is possibly the most obscure poison ever used. It was first discovered by the Polish-French scientist Marie Curie and her husband Pierre in 1898 and named after her country of origin, Poland. Litvinenko is the only confirmed victim recorded, although there have been allegations that it may have also been used to kill the Palestinian leader Yasser Arafat. It is highly toxic—the fatal dose is estimated to be a millionth of a gram—but the victim needs to take it internally, and it has a short shelf life.

failed to improve, he was taken to London's University College Hospital. Doctors believed that he had been poisoned—by this time he was being kept under police guard—but they couldn't discover what the poison was. Could it be thallium? The symptoms largely seemed to fit, in particular the catastrophic reduction in his white blood cells, and the toxic heavy metal was not so hard to find for those with the right connections—it had been a key component of rat poison in the past. However, there were contradictions—Litvinenko was not suffering from the numbness of the extremities, which is a key symptom of thallium poisoning.

Litvinenko was interviewed by police officers for a total of nearly nine hours; despite his deteriorating condition, he was determined to tell his story. News had reached the press, and the hospital was besieged by journalists. A Russian agent poisoned by mysterious assassins in the middle of London was a sensational story. On November 20, a shocking picture was authorized to appear in the media. A man who had always prided himself on his fitness, Litvinenko was shown in bed, bald, yellow with jaundice, and surrounded by wires and beeping machines. If anyone had doubted it before, the image made it clear that he was dying. Asked for comment on the allegation that Litvinenko had been poisoned by Russian agents, the Kremlin issued an official denial of any involvement. Litvinenko's wife and son were summoned to the hospital in the middle of the night on November 23, only to be told on their arrival that he had died a short time earlier.

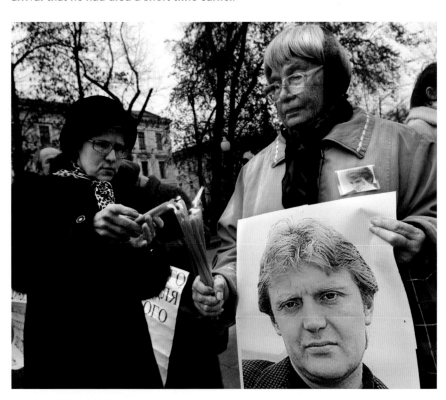

After the death. *Human rights activists held demonstrations against the assassination of Litvinenko in both Moscow and London.*

TRACKING THE POLONIUM TRAIL

A couple of days after Alexander Litvinenko's death, British government scientists finally discovered what had poisoned him. Tests at the UK Atomic Weapons Establishment at Aldermaston, Berkshire, Britain's highly secretive chemical research facility, found polonium 210, an extraordinarily rare substance, in a urine sample. It can only be produced in a nuclear reactor. It is readily absorbed into all sorts of substances and can only poison a person if swallowed. Once inside the body, though, it is a certain killer.

Now that the police knew what they were looking for, they could track it. Scaramella, who had briefly been a suspect, was now dropped from the inquiry altogether. Scientists began to uncover a polonium trail stretching all over London and beyond. Before his meeting with Lugovoi and Kovtun, Litvinenko had been "clean" and left no traces; after it, everywhere he had subsequently gone was contaminated with polonium. When tested, traces of it were found gleaming on the surfaces in Lugovoi and Kovtun's hotel rooms, in the bathrooms and the bar at the Millennium, and everywhere the pair had been subsequently—even at the Emirates Stadium, where Lugovoi had watched soccer with his family. The wealth of evidence was beginning to stack up.

By the time there was concrete evidence of the crime, the two Russians were long gone. The Kremlin dismissed the story as fantasy, and refused even to discuss extradition. Litvinenko, on his deathbed, had squarely accused the Kremlin and, specifically, Vladimir Putin, of arranging his assassination—and an official inquiry held in London ten years after his death would say that the operation to kill Litvinenko was "probably approved" by the head of the FSB and by President Putin—but there would be no trial and no conviction for his murder.

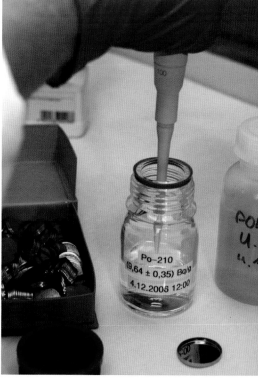

Testing for polonium.
Polonium is so rare that even scientists at Aldermaston, Britain's top-secret chemical research facility, had problems identifying it. Once it had been identified, though, it tied the poisoning closely to Russia.

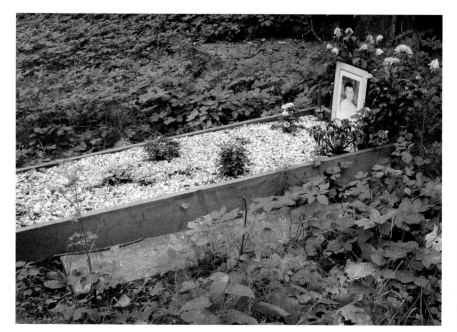

Uneasy bedfellows. *On December 8, 2006, Alexander Litvinenko was buried in the iconic Highgate Cemetery in North London. Ironically, the cemetery is also the resting place of, among other eminent figures, Karl Marx.*

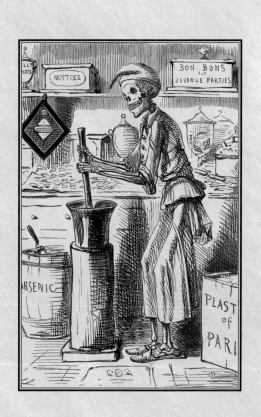

INDEX

Page numbers in **bold** indicate main entries; page numbers in *italics* indicate illustrations.

Canadian Medical Association Journal, 88

Canidia, 7, **30–31**

cantarella, 11, 55

cantharidin (Spanish fly), 11, 75

Cappelle, Marie, *see* Lafarge, Marie

Carina, Rose, 123

Carroll, Lieutenant Gary, 107

Carter, Edwin, *see* Litvinenko, Alexander

Cassius, Dio, 35

Castellesi, Adriano, 55

castor oil plant (*Ricinus communis*), 154, *154*; *see also* ricin

Catherine of Aragon, 47–51

"Catherine wheel" (torture), 62

dei Cattanei, Vannozza, 54

chambre ardente, 64, 65

Charenton Asylum, France, 76, 77

Charles IX, king of France, 44, 45

Charles V, Holy Roman Emperor, 48

"La Chaussée," 62

chemical warfare, **136–43**, *137*; *see also* poison gas

Chemical Weapons Convention (1997), 141, 142, 143

Chernobyl nuclear disaster, 174

Chiba, Japan, 161

Chicago, Illinois, 86–7

chloracne, 175, 177

chlorine gas, 137–8, 139, 142, 143

Christie, Agatha, 18, 100

Claudius, Roman emperor, 28–30, 35

Clement VII, Pope, 43

Cleopatra VII Philopator, pharaoh of Egypt, 6, **20–25**, *21, 22, 24, 25*

Cleopatra Selene, 23

Cleopatra Testing Poisons on Condemned Men (Cabanel), 25, *25*

Clover, Matilda, 85, 88–9

Cold War, 142, 153

Coldwater, Michigan, 109

Collard, Monsieur, 91

Columbus, Christopher, 39, 41

Commission, The (Mafia governing body), 157

de Condé, Caroline, Princesse, 73

conquistadors, 39

Conspiracy of Amboise, 44

Cotton, Frederick, 98

Cotton, Margaret, 98

Cotton, Mary Ann, 8, 9, **98–101**, *97, 101*

Cranstoun, William Henry, 67–71

Cream, Dr Thomas Neill, **86–9**, *85*

Cream, William, 87

Crippen, Cora, 110–12, *110*

Crippen, Dr Hawley Harvey, 8–9, **108–13**, *109, 112, 113*

Crippen, Myron and Andresse, 109

Crito (Plato), 18, 19

crocus, 35

Cuba, 41

Curie, Marie and Pierre, 182

Curwen, Bennett, 50

cyanide, 11, 28, 117, 118, 138, 140, 150, 158

D

Dabin, Jean, 134

daimonion, 15, 16, 17

Dali, Salvador, 77

Damascus, Syria, 142

Darzhavna Sigurnost (Bulgarian secret service) 155

deadly nightshade, 28, 35

DeCavalcante family, 157, 158

Degesch (Deutsche Gesellschaft für Schädlingsbekämpfung mbH), 139

Democratic Republic of the Congo, 163

Dendera Temple, Egypt, *22*

Deron, Dr Henri, 134

Dew, Chief Inspector Walter, 111–13

"Diamond Circle Club," 130

dianisidine chlorosulfate, 137

Dioscorides 31

dioxin, 9, 11, 141, 175, *175*, 177

Donneybrook Medical Centre, Hyde, 169, *169*

Donworth, Ellen, 88

Doss, Nancy "Nannie," 9, **126–31**, *127, 128, 129, 131*

Doss, Samuel 127, 130–31

Douma, Syria, 143

Drouet Institute for the Deaf, 110

Drusus, 34

Dundee Courier, 101

E

Edinburgh, Scotland, 86

Edward IV, king of England, 47

Edward VI, king of England, 51

Edward, Charles, 98, 100–101

Egerton, Stan, 168, 170

Egypt, 21–5

electric chair, *124*, 125

Elizabeth I, queen of England, 51

Elizabeth of York, 47

Elmore, Belle, *see* Crippen, Cora

Emirates Stadium, 183

Epodes (Horace), 31

d'Este, Alfonso, 54

Ethiopia, 143

Exili (Nicolò Egidi), 61

F

Faulkner, Mary Ann, 86

Favato, Carina, 124

Ferdinand, king of Spain, 39, 41

fig (*Ficus carica*) 35, *35*

First Sacred War (595–585 BC), 143

Fisher, Bishop John, 7, 49–51, *50, 51*

Flanner, Janet, 134

Florence, Italy, 43

Florida, 40, 41

de la Fontanges, Duchesse (Marie Angelique de Scorailles), 65

food tasting, 29, 35, 63

Forbes, Judge John, 170

forensic science, 8

Fort Lauderdale, Florida, 106

Fountain of Youth, 40–41

France, 8, 9, 43–5, 61–5, 81, 91–5, 133–5, 137, 143

Francis I, king of France, 43, 64

Francis II, king of France, 43–4

Franco-Prussian War (1870–71), 81

Frazier, Huey and Lucille, 103, 104

French, Sir John, 137

"French school of poisoners," 44

French Wars of Religion (1562–98), 44

FSB (successor agency of KGB), 179, 183

Fumihiro, Jōyū, 164

G

Galba, Roman emperor, 30

Garat, Madame, 91–2

Gardener, Kate, 86

Gardner, Gerald, 43

gas, *see* poison gas

gastric fever, 100

Geneva Protocol (1925), 143

Genghis Khan, 173

Genovese family, 158

Germanicus, 31

Germany, 137–40, 142

Philadelphia, Pennsylvania, 121–5
    Philadelphia Poison Ring, 8,
        120–25
phosgene gas, 138, 143
Pinturicchio, Il, 54
Plataea, Greece, 143
Plato, 17, 18, 19
Pliny the Elder, 31
Plutarch 22, 23, 24, 25
plutonium, 155
poison gas 137–8
    chlorine gas, 137–8, 139, 142, 143
    dianisidine chlorosulfate, 137
    gas masks, *10, 137*
    mustard gas, 137, 138, 142, 143
    phosgene gas, 138, 143
    xylyl bromide, 137
    Zyklon B, 10, 138–9, *138*
poisons
    abrin, 155
    aconite (*Aconitum napellus*), 11, *11*,
        28, 83, *83*
    Aqua Tofana, 7, 11, 63
    arsenic, 11, 69, 93, *93*, 99, 100, 104,
        105, 123–4, 129
    cantarella, 11, 55
    cantharidin (Spanish fly), 11, 75
    castor oil plant (*Ricinus communis*),
        154, *154*
    cyanide, 11, 28, 117, 118, 138, 140,
        150, 158
    deadly nightshade, 28, 35
    dioxin, 9, 11, 141, 175, *175*, 177
    hemlock (*Conium maculatum*), 11,
        11, 18, *18*, 28, 35
    henbane (*Hyoscyamus niger*), 11, *11*,
        28, *28*
    hyoscine (*Hyoscine hydrobromide*), 11,
        111, 112, 113
    manchineel (*Hippomane mancinella*),
        11, *11*, 40, 41, *41*
    mandrake, 28
    morphine, 11, 82–3, 167, 170
    mushrooms, 29
    polonium, 9, 11, 181, 182, 183, *183*
    ricin, 11, 154, 155
    rosary pea (*Abrus precatorius*), 155
    snake bites. 24
    strychnine (*Strychnos nux-vomica*),
        11, 28, 86
    thallium, 182
    yew extract, 28, 35
    see also poison gas; nerve agents

de Poitiers, Diane, 43
Pokrovskoye, Siberia, 115
Poland, 182
polonium, 9, 11, 181, 182, 183, *183*
Ponce de Léon, Juan, 7, **38–41**, *39, 40*
Pontier, Emma 93, 94
Port Kaituma, Guyana, 150
Porton Down, 154, 155
Postumus, 35
Prince, The (Machiavelli), 54, 57
Prussia, 81
Ptolemy I Soter, pharaoh of Egypt, 21
Ptolemy Philadelphus, 23
Ptolemy XII Auletes, pharaoh of
    Egypt, 21
Ptolemy XIII, pharaoh of Egypt, 22
Ptolemy XIV, pharaoh of Egypt, 22
Puerto Rico, 40–41
Purishkevich, Vladimir, 118
Putin, Vladimir, 179, 180, 183

Q

quail, 18
Quebec, Canada, 85, 112
Quesnet, Marie-Constance, 77
Quick-Manning, John, 98, 101

R

Racine, Jean, 30
Radio Free Europe, 153
Raikes, Thomas, 95
Rasputin (Grigori Yefimovich Novykh),
    9, **114–19**, *115, 117, 119*
Redwood Valley, California, 148–9
Reformation, 43
Reinsch test, 8, 101
Richmond, Indiana, 147
ricin, 11, 154, 155; *see also* castor oil
    plant
Riley, Thomas, 101
Robinson, James, 97–8
Robson, Mary Ann, *see* Cotton,
    Mary Ann
Roman Empire, 6–7, 22–4, 27–31,
    33–5
Romanov dynasty, 116
Romauldo, Josephine, 125
Rome, Italy, 53–6
Rommel, Field Marshal Erwin, 140
Roose, Richard, 50–51
rosary pea (*Abrus precatorius*), 155
Rudolfinerhaus, Vienna, 175, 176, 177
Rue de Madagascar, Paris, 133, *134*

Russia, 9–10, 115–19, 137, 161, 163,
    165, 173, 179–83
Russian Orthodox Church, 115–16, 161
    Khlysty sect, 116
Russo-Turkish War (1877–78) 81
Ryan, Leo J, 150

S

de Sade, Abbé, 73
de Sade, Louis-Marie, 74
de Sade, Marquis (Donatien Alphonse
    François), 8, **72–7**, *73, 76*
St Bartholomew's Day Massacre
    (1572), *44*, 45
St James' Hospital, London, 153–4
St Petersburg, Russia, 116, 117
Saint Seraphim, 116
Saint-Simon, (Louis de Rouvroy,
    Duc de Saint-Simon), 65
de Sainte-Croix, Jean-Baptiste Godin,
    61–2
San Francisco Examiner, 148
San José Church, Old San Juan,
    Puerto Rico, 41
San Juan Bautista Cathedral, Puerto
    Rico, 41, *41*
Santa Maria della Febbre Church,
    Rome, 57
Santervás de Campos, Spain, 39
Saratoga, New York, 89
sarin, 10, 11, 141, 142, 143, 163–4
Sarov, Russia, 116
Saumane-de-Vaucluse, Auvergne,
    73
Scaramella, Mario, 180, 183
Schecter, Arnold, 177
Schrader, Gerhard, 143
Scribonia, 33–4
Scribonius Largus, 31
Selassie, Haile, 143
Sertürner, Friedrich, 82
Seven Years' War (1756–63), 73
Seymour, Jane, 51
Sforza, Giovanni, 54, 55
Shakespeare, William, 21, 24
Shinto (religion), 161
Shipman, Harold Frederick, 8–9,
    166–71, *167, 168*
Shipman, Primrose, 168–9
Shrivell, Emma, 89
Sicily, Italy, 157
Simenon, Georges, 135
snake bites, 24

REFERENCES

Socrates
Bettany Hughes, *The Hemlock Cup: Socrates, Athens and the Search for the Good Life* (Vintage, 2011)

Cleopatra
Joyce Tyldesley, *Cleopatra: Last Queen of Egypt* (Profile Books, 2009)

Locusta, Canidia, and Martina; Livia
Thomas Wiedemann, *The Julio-Claudian Emperors* (Bristol Classical Press, 1991)

Juan Ponce de León
Robert H. Fuson, *Juan Ponce de Léon and the Spanish Discovery of Puerto Rico and Florida* (McDonald and Woodward, 1999)
www.mnn.com/family/protection-safety/blogs/why-manchineel-might-be-earths-most-dangerous-tree

Catherine de' Medici
Geoffrey Treasure, *The Huguenots* (Yale University Press, 2013)
www.britannica.com/biography/Catherine-de-Medici

Poisoning at the Tudor Court
Elizabeth Norton, *Anne Boleyn: Henry VIII's Obsession* (Amberley Publishing, 2009)
englishhistoryauthors.blogspot.com/2014/07/the-death-of-bishops-poisoner.html

The Borgias
Christopher Hibbert, *The Borgias* (Constable, 2011)
Mary Hollingsworth, *The Borgias: History's Most Notorious Dynasty* (Quercus, 2014)

The Affair of the Poisons
Somerset, Anne, *The Affair of the Poisons* (Weidenfeld & Nicholson, 2003)
History of the Chateau de Versailles:
en.chateauversailles.fr/discover/history

Mary Blandy
William Roughead, *The Trial of Mary Blandy* (online at Gutenberg.org, 1914)

Marquis de Sade
Neil Schaeffer, *The Marquis de Sade: A Life* (Hamish Hamilton, 1999)

George Henry Lamson
Adam, Hargrave L., *Trial of George Henry Lamson* (W. Hodge & Co, 1913)

Thomas Cream
James H Hodge, ed, *Famous Trials 5*, including the trial of Dr Thomas Neill Cream (Penguin, 1994)

Mary Ann Cotton
www.britannica.com/biography/Mary-Ann-Cotton

Audrey Marie Hilley
Philip E Ginsberg, *Poisoned Blood: The True Story of Marie Hilley, Cold-Blooded Killer* (Michael O'Mara Books, 1993)

Dr Crippen
Harry Hodge ed, *Famous Trials 1*, including the trial of Dr Harvey Hawley Crippen (Penguin, 1994)

Rasputin
Frances Welch, *Rasputin: A Short Life* (Simon & Schuster, 2014)
www.smithsonianmag.com/history/murder-rasputin-100-years-later-180961572/

The Philadelphia Poison Ring
George Cooper, *Poison Widows: A True Story of Witchcraft, Arsenic, and Murder* (St Martins Press, 1999)
philadelphiaencyclopedia.org/archive/great-depression/

Nannie Doss
Charles Montaldo, www.thoughtco.com/serial-killer-nannie-doss-973101
Gordon Harvey, http://www.encyclopediaofalabama.org/article/h-3619

Violette Nozière
Sarah Maza, *Violette Nozière A Story of Murder in 1930s Paris* (University of California Press, 2011)

Poisons in Warfare
www.britannica.com/topic/Defining-Weapons-of-Mass-Destruction-917325
www.bbc.co.uk/news/magazine-31042472

The Rev Jim Jones
Jeff Guinn, *The Road to Jonestown: Jim Jones and the Peoples Temple* (Simon & Schuster, 2017)

Georgi Markov
Nick Paton Walsh, "Markov's umbrella assassin revealed" (*The Guardian*, June 6, 2005)

Richard Kuklinski
www.nytimes.com/2006/03/09/nyregion/richard-kuklinski-70-a-killer-of-many-people-and-many-ways-dies.html

The Tokyo Subway Sarin Poisonings
www.bbc.co.uk/news/world-asia-35975069

Victor Yushchenko
www.newscientist.com/article/dn17570-skin-growths-saved-poisoned-ukrainian-president/

Alexander Litvinenko
Esther Addley, "Alexander Litvinenko told Met police Putin ordered his murder, inquiry told" (*The Guardian*, January 27, 2015)
Oliver Bullough, "The story of how Russia killed a spy on UK soil" (GQ *Magazine*, March 7, 2018)

Official Reports
The British government's enquiries into the crimes of Harold Shipman and the murder of Alexander Litvinenko are available online. Both are highly detailed and engrossing reads. Both can be found at assets.publishing.service.gov.uk.
The Shipman Inquiry: in 6 parts, published between 2002 and 2005
The Litvinenko Inquiry: published 2016

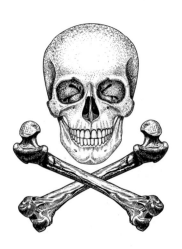